Controlling Diabetes Naturally

with
Chinese Medicine

Lynn M. Kuchinski

BLUE POPPY PRESS

Published by:

BLUE POPPY PRESS
A Division of Blue Poppy Enterprises, Inc.
3450 Penrose Place, Suite 110
BOULDER, CO 80301

First Edition, September, 1999
ISBN 1-891845-06-3 LC# 99-72726

COMP Designation: Original work
Printed at Johnson Printing in Boulder, CO

10 9 8 7 6 5 4 3 2 1

Other books in this series include:
Curing Insomnia Naturally with Chinese Medicine
Curing Hay Fever Naturally with Chinese Medicine
Curing Headaches Naturally with Chinese Medicine
Better Breast Health Naturally with Chinese Medicine
Curing Depression Naturally with Chinese Medicine
Curing Arthritis Naturally with Chinese Medicine
Curing PMS Naturally with Chinese Medicine
Managing Menopause Naturally with Chinese Medicine

Preface

Diabetes is on the rise throughout the world in developing nations, and diabetes can affect a person's life in profound ways. Currently, the annual economic cost of diabetes in the United States alone is over $92 billion. Countries with a traditionally low rate of diabetes are now experiencing an increase in the incidence of diabetes along with the importation of the Western diet and high sugar, fast food restaurants. Although diabetes is an ever increasing threat, it does not have to occur. When it does, Chinese medicine has ways to cure or alleviate it.

The stress and dietary irregularities of our Western lifestyle are a virtual breeding ground for imbalance, disorder, and disease. As a practitioner of Chinese medicine in the United States, I see patients every day who exhibit the symptoms of hypoglycemia, the precursor of diabetes. Sometimes these symptoms are associated with other disorders, but most often they are directly associated with the condition that leads to diabetes and its devastating effect on our lives.

With this book, I hope to call attention to the fact that Chinese medicine, *i.e.*, acupuncture and especially Chinese medicinals, offers a remedy to the gradual decline that diabetics commonly suffer. Chinese medicine not only alleviates the symptoms of diabetes but also actually helps lower blood and urine sugar levels, thus allowing diabetics the opportunity to live without constant dependence on insulin. This may sound like a tall order, but the Chinese medical literature proves that Chinese medicine along with proper diet and lifestyle modifications does offer this possibility. Hopefully, this book will encourage diabetics and their families to venture into the world of Chinese medicine to see what it has to offer.

In the West, we are not usually counseled by our medical practitioners on how to make the changes in our lives that are necessary to maintain good health. Chinese medicine, on the other hand, can help with suggestions on exercise and relaxation. It can also help patients control and curb their desire for sugar and other foods associated with pre-diabetic conditions. Chinese medicine does this by treating with acupuncture and so-called Chinese herbal medicine. In addition, it has a rich history of counseling in dietary recommendations. When these methods of treatment are combined, the results are powerful, and patients, by participating in their own therapy, are enabled to reclaim their own health.

Each of us probably knows someone who is suffering from diabetes. This is a disease that touches most of us, our families, and our friends. When left unattended or when treated with routine Western standards, the diabetic is faced with possible degeneration and complications with the kidneys, heart, vision, and nervous system. It is my hope that the basic information in this book will introduce Chinese medicine to readers who may not know about it and that, for some at least, the process of degeneration will be halted. If this book can accomplish that, then it will have served its purpose.

Thanks are due to Bob Flaws for allowing me to use so much of his material from other *Curing* books in this series and for his furnishing me Chinese research materials on this disease. Without his help and encouragement, I could not have created this book.

Lynn M. Kuchinski
Albuquerque, NM
October, 1998

Contents

Preface

Introduction

Joanne had been feeling badly all week, but today was the worst yet. This morning she could hardly get out of bed. Since she was running late to work, she stopped to pick up some doughnuts and coffee and ate those in the car on the way to the office. She had meetings all morning which ran right through lunchtime; so she finished the doughnuts, had another coffee, and stopped at the vending machine for an apple pie and candy bar. By 3:00 P.M. at her desk, she was so tired she could hardly move, pale, sweating, and weak in the limbs. Heart palpitations made her anxious and irritable. How could she be so weak and without energy? After all, she had a lot of sugar today to boost her energy. The last six months had been like today, and she didn't know how much more she could tolerate. The sugar cravings seemed to run her life, yet the more she gave in to the cravings, the more her days were out of control. Now, at the end of the day, with a migraine coming on, the future didn't look very bright.

Sound familiar? If so, this book may very well help you break the cycle of diabetes. Traditional Chinese doctors have been treating diabetes safely and effectively for tens of centuries.

This book is a layperson's guide to the diagnosis and treatment of diabetes with Chinese medicine. In it, you will learn what causes diabetes and what you can do about it. Hopefully, you will be able to identify yourself and your symptoms in these pages. If you can see yourself in the signs and symptoms I discuss below, I feel confident I will be able to share with you a number of self-help techniques which can minimize your discomfort. Chinese medicine cannot cure every disease, but when it comes to diabetes, Chinese medicine is the best alternative I know. When someone calls me and says that diabetes is their major complaint, I know that, if they follow my advice, together we can cure or at least reduce the difficult symptoms.

What is hypoglycemia?

Hypoglycemia is a condition where the sugar level in the blood is abnormally low, less than 50mg/dl (milligrams of glucose per deciliter of blood). Hypoglycemia in Greek literally means low blood sugar (*hypo* = under or low, *glykys* = sweet, *haima* = blood). The normal range for blood sugar is 60-120 mg/dl depending on when a person has eaten last. Most individuals who are hypoglycemic actually fluctuate between low and high blood sugar levels. Hypoglycemia is a common symptom and may be associated with a number of other diseases, the most common of these is diabetes.

How does the body control glucose?

The amount of glucose in the blood is controlled primarily by the two hormones, insulin and glucagon. Too much or too little of these two hormones can cause the blood sugar levels to drop too low (hypoglycemia) or rise too high (hyperglycemia). Cortisol, growth hormone, and catecholamines (epinephrine and norepinephrine) can also influence the blood sugar levels. The pancreas, a gland in the upper abdomen, produces both insulin and glucagon. The pancreas contains a hormone-producing tissue called the islets of Langerhans. When blood sugar levels rise after a meal, the beta cells in the islets of Langerhans release insulin. The insulin helps glucose enter the body cells, lowering the blood levels of glucose to the normal range. When blood sugar falls too low, the alpha cells, also located in the islets of Langerhans, secrete glucagon. This triggers the liver to release stored glycogen and change it into glucose, thus raising blood sugar levels to the normal range. The body's muscles also store glycogen and can be called upon to convert that glycogen into glucose.

Causes of hypoglycemia

The most common of all hypoglycemias is called functional reactive hypoglycemia. When complex carbohydrates are eaten, the body breaks them down gradually and the basic sugars resulting from this process are slowly released into the bloodstream. In the bloodstream, these sugars circulate as energy for the brain and body organs. The brain alone will utilize up to 80% of the circulating blood sugar. However, when simple carbohydrates, like refined sugar and flour products, are consumed habitually, the body quickly digests them and then floods the bloodstream with glucose. The pancreatic beta cells must respond again and again to this excessive level of blood sugar in order to bring the sugar into the body's cells. Excess sugar in the bloodstream is stored in three locations. In the liver, it is stored as glycogen; in the fat cells, it is converted to adipose; and in the muscles, it is converted to muscle glycogen. When this happens, the blood sugar levels drop severely, and that information is fed back to the hypothalamus, pituitary, and thyroid glands. During this time, the symptoms of hypoglycemia become apparent, as discussed below. These glands then communicate to the liver that the stored glycogen must be changed back into sugar and released into the bloodstream to raise the blood sugar levels.

In this way the body makes an heroic attempt to replace and balance the blood sugar levels. Unfortunately, if the body must constantly send out insulin to balance the effect of a simple carbohydrate meal or snack, the pancreas and other organs will suffer. And when the burden constantly falls on the adrenals, pituitary, and liver to counterbalance the aftereffects, these organs will suffer depletion as well.

The signs & symptoms of hypoglycemia

A person with hypoglycemia may feel weak, drowsy, confused, hungry, and dizzy. They may have pale complexions and may suffer from headaches, sweating, rapid heartbeat, and feel cold

3

and clammy. They might suffer from heart palpitations, tremors and shaking, and may be very irritable. There could be vision problems, anxiety and nervousness, palsy, and lack of muscle coordination. In severe cases, there may be personality disturbances, loss of consciousness, convulsions, and coma. Many times, these people feel that their energy is chronically low and that they need to eat sugar throughout the day as the only way to relieve their symptoms. Severe hypoglycemia can be close to insulin shock and is considered a medical emergency.

How Western medicine treats hypoglycemia

When Western MDs try to treat hypoglycemia, they usually do so by prescribing oral glucose or sucrose to be taken when the symptoms of diabetes appear, or take 2-3 tablespoons of sugar in fruit juice or water. They may also suggest that the patient relieve their emotional stress, get more exercise, and eat a protein rich, high complex carbohydrate diet.

While counseling the hypoglycemic patient on exercise and dietary change is necessary for controlling the blood sugar levels, it is the baseline recommendation that Chinese medical practitioners give, not only for diabetes but also for all other disorders as well. What we eat, how we use our bodies, and how we handle our emotions stand at the forefront in regaining and keeping our health and well-being. Most sufferers of hypo-glycemia and diabetes are already on a rollercoaster of high and low blood sugar levels, with day-long sugar cravings that actually worsen their symptoms longterm. Recommending that the patient take more sugar by adding to fruit juice or by glucose tablets only serves to promote the cycle of high and low blood sugar levels and causes the body's organs to respond even more dramatically in an attempt to balance the blood sugar. Keep in mind that the average adult has one to two teaspoons of blood sugar circulating in the body at any one time, with a smaller amount stored in the liver for emergency use. Eating 4 oz of chocolate cake with icing (10 teaspoons of sugar) and a 6 oz soda (3 teaspoons of sugar) will cause sugar overload chaos in the body. The body then must bring the blood sugar level down by means of the complicated mechanism that has been described above. Eating that much sugar at a time can cause the pancreas to produce too much insulin which, in turn, brings the blood sugar level below normal, causing the symptoms which we have already discussed. Taking more refined sugar at this time is like pouring gasoline on a fire.

So what is diabetes?

Diabetes is actually a condition of hyperglycemia. Remember earlier we discussed how the body must handle simple carbohydrates, like refined sugar and flour products, when they are consumed habitually. The body quickly digests them and then floods the bloodstream with glucose. The pancreatic beta cells must respond again and again to this excessive level of blood sugar in order to bring the sugar into the body's cells. When this happens, the blood sugar levels drop severely, and that information is fed back to the hypothalamus, pituitary, and thyroid glands. During this time, the symptoms of hypoglycemia become apparent, as we have already discussed. These glands then communicate to the liver that the stored glycogen must be changed back into sugar and released into the bloodstream to raise the blood sugar levels. In this way, the body attempts again and again to replace and balance the blood sugar levels. Unfortunately, if the body must constantly send out insulin to balance the effect of a simple carbohydrate meal or snack, the pancreas and other organs will suffer. And when the burden constantly falls on the adrenals, pituitary, and liver to counterbalance the after effects, these organs will suffer depletion as well. Diabetes actually happens when the body cannot use glucose for fuel because either the pancreas has broken down and is not able to make enough insulin or the insulin that is available is not effective.

How Western medicine treats diabetes

Western medicine aims at lowering blood sugar levels by prescribing insulin or oral drugs. However, too much insulin or irregular eating habits can cause hypoglycemia in diabetics and is referred to as "insulin reaction." In addition, if insulin is discontinued, the blood sugar levels will immediately rise and even the long term use of insulin will not prevent other diabetic complications, such as renal failure, neuropathy, retinopathy, and cardiac distress.

Happily, Chinese medicine has a number of safe and effective, low cost and non-addictive alternatives which have been used in Asia for hundreds and thousands of years.

East is East and West is West

In order for the reader to understand and make sense of the rest of this book on Chinese medicine and diabetes, one must understand that Chinese medicine is a distinct and separate system of medical thought and practice from modern Western medicine. This means that one must shift models of reality when it comes to thinking about Chinese medicine. It has taken the Chinese more than 2,000 years to develop this medical system. In fact, Chinese medicine is the oldest continually practiced, literate, professional medicine in the world. As such, one cannot understand Chinese medicine by trying to explain it in Western scientific or medical terms.

Most people reading this book have probably taken high school biology back when they were sophomores. Whether we recognize it or not, most of us Westerners think of what we learned about the human body in high school as "the really real" description of reality, not one possible description. However, if Chinese medicine is to make any sense to Westerners at all, one must be able to entertain the notion that there are potentially other valid descriptions of the human body, its functions, health, and disease.

6

In grappling with this fundamentally important issue, it is useful to think about the concepts of a map and the terrain it describes.

If we take the United States of America as an example, we can have numerous different maps of this country's land mass. One map might show population. Another might show per capita incomes. Another might show religious or ethnic distributions. Yet another might be a road map. And still another might be a map showing political, *i.e.*, state boundaries. In fact, there could be an infinite number of potentially different maps of the United States depending on what one was trying to show and do. As long as the map is based on accurate information and has been created with self-consistent logic, then one map is not necessarily more correct than another. The issue is to use the right map for what you are trying to do. If one wants to drive from Chicago to Washington DC, then a road map is probably the right one for that job but is not necessarily a truer or "more real" description of the United States than a map showing annual rainfall.

What I am getting at here is that the map is *not* the terrain. The Western biological map of the human body is only one potentially useful medical map. It is no more true than the traditional Chinese medical map, and the "facts" of one map cannot be reduced to the criteria or standards of another unless they share the same logic right from the beginning. As long as the Western medical map is capable of solving a person's disease in a cost-effective, time-efficient manner without side effects or iatrogenesis (meaning doctor-caused disease), then it is a useful map. Chinese medicine needs to be judged in the same way. The Chinese medical map of health and disease is just as "real" as the Western biological map as long as, using it, professional practitioners are able to solve their patients' health problems in a safe and effective way.

Therefore, the following chapter is an introduction to the basics of Chinese medicine. Unless one understands some of the fundamental theories and "facts" of Chinese medicine, one will not be able to understand or accept the reasons for some of the Chinese medical treatments of diabetes. As the reader will quickly see from this brief overview of Chinese medicine, "This doesn't look like Kansas, Toto!"

An Overview of the Chinese Medical Map

In this chapter, we will look at an overview of Chinese medicine. In particular, we will discuss yin and yang, qi, blood, and essence, the viscera and bowels, and the channels and network vessels. In the following chapter, we will go on to see how Chinese medicine views diabetes. After that, we will look at the Chinese medical diagnosis and treatment of the various patterns of diabetes identified by professional practitioners of Chinese medicine.

Yin & Yang

To understand Chinese medicine, one must first understand the concepts of yin and yang since these are the most basic concepts in this system. Yin and yang are the cornerstones for understanding, diagnosing, and treating the body and mind in Chinese medicine. In a sense, all the other theories and concepts of Chinese medicine are nothing other than an elaboration of yin and yang. Most people have probably already heard of yin and yang but may have only a fuzzy idea of what these terms mean.

The concepts of yin and yang can be used to describe everything that exists in the universe, including all the parts and functions of the body. Originally, yin referred to the shady side of a hill and yang to the sunny side of the hill. Since sunshine and shade are two, interdependent sides of a single reality, these two aspects of the hill are seen as part of a single whole. Other examples of yin and yang are that night exists only in relation to day and cold exists only in relation to heat. According to Chinese thought, every single thing that exists in the universe has these two aspects, a yin and a yang. Thus everything has a front and a back, a top and a bottom, a left and a right, and a beginning and an end. However, a thing is yin or yang only in relation to its paired complement. Nothing is in itself yin or yang.

It is the concepts of yin and yang which make Chinese medicine a holistic medicine. This is because, based on this unitary and complementary vision of reality, no body part or body function is viewed as separate or isolated from the whole person. The table below shows a partial list of yin and yang pairs as they apply to the body.

Yin	Yang
form	function
organs	bowels
blood	qi
inside	outside
front of body	back of body
right side	left side
lower body	upper body
cool, cold	warm, hot
stillness	activity, movement

However, it is important to remember that each item listed is either yin or yang only in relation to its complementary partner. Nothing is absolutely and all by itself either yin or yang. As we can see from the above list, it is possible to describe every aspect of the body in terms of yin and yang.

Qi

Qi (pronounced chee) and blood are the two most important complementary pairs of yin and yang within the human body. It is said that, in the world, yin and yang are water and fire, but in the human body, yin and yang are blood and qi. Qi is yang in relation to blood which is yin. Qi is often translated as energy and certainly energy is a manifestation of qi. Chinese language scholars would say, however, that qi is larger than any single type of energy described by modern Western science. Paul Unschuld, perhaps the greatest living sinologist, translates the word qi as influences. This conveys the sense that qi is what is responsible for change and movement. Thus, within Chinese medicine, qi is that which motivates all movement and transformation or change.

In Chinese medicine, qi is defined as having five specific functions:

1. Defense
It is qi which is responsible for protecting the exterior of the body from invasion by external pathogens. This qi, called defensive qi, flows through the exterior portion of the body.

2. Transformation
Qi transforms substances so that they can be utilized by the body. An example of this function is the transformation of the food we eat into nutrients to nourish the body, thus producing more qi and blood.

3. Warming
Qi, being relatively yang, is inherently warm and one of the main functions of the qi is to warm the entire body, both inside and out. If this warming function of the qi is weak, cold may cause the flow of qi and blood to be congealed similar to cold's effect on water producing ice.

4. Restraint
It is qi which holds all the organs and substances in their proper place. Thus all the organs, blood, and fluids need qi to keep them from falling or leaking out of their specific pathways. If this

function of the qi is weak, then problems like uterine prolapse, easy bruising, or urinary incontinence may occur.

5. Transportation
Qi provides the motivating force for all transportation and movement in the body. Every aspect of the body that moves is moved by the qi. Hence the qi moves the blood and body fluids throughout the body. It moves food through the stomach and blood through the vessels.

Blood

In Chinese medicine, blood refers to the red fluid that flows through our vessels the same as in modern Western medicine, but it also has meanings and implications which are different from those in modern Western medicine. Most basically, blood is that substance which nourishes and moistens all the body tissues. Without blood, no body tissue can function properly. In addition, when blood is insufficient or scanty, tissue becomes dry and withers.

Qi and blood are closely interrelated. It is said that, "Qi is the commander of the blood and blood is the mother of qi." This means that it is qi which moves the blood but that it is the blood which provides the nourishment and physical foundation for the creation and existence of the qi.

In Chinese medicine, blood provides the following functions for the body:

1. Nourishment
Blood nourishes the body. Along with qi, the blood goes to every part of the body. When the blood is insufficient, function decreases and tissue atrophies or shrinks.

2. Moistening
Blood moistens the body tissues. This includes the skin, eyes, and ligaments and tendons or what are simply called the sinews in

Chinese medicine. Thus blood insufficiency can cause drying out and consequent stiffening of various body tissues throughout the body.

3. Blood provides the material foundation for the spirit or mind.

In Chinese medicine, the mind and body are not two separate things. The spirit is nothing other than a great accumulation of qi. The blood (yin) supplies the material support and nourishment for the spirit (yang) so that it accumulates, becomes bright (*i.e.*, conscious and clever), and stays rooted in the body. If the blood becomes insufficient, the mind can "float," causing problems like insomnia, agitation, and unrest.

Essence

Along with qi and blood, essence is one of the three most important constituents of the body. Essence is the most fundamental, essential material the body utilizes for its growth, maturation, and reproduction. There are two forms of this essence. We inherit essence from our parents and we also produce our own essence from the food we eat, the liquids we drink, and the air we breathe.

The essence which comes from our parents is what determines our basic constitution, strength, and vitality. We each have a finite, limited amount of this inherited essence. It is important to protect and conserve this essence because all bodily functions depend upon it and, when it is gone, we die. Thus the depletion of essence has serious implications for our overall health and well-being. Happily, the essence derived from food and drink helps to bolster and support this inherited essence. Thus, if we eat well and do not consume more qi and blood than we create each day, then when we sleep at night, this surplus qi and more especially blood is transformed into essence.

The Viscera & Bowels

In Chinese medicine, the internal organs (called viscera so as not to become confused with the Western biological entities of the same name) have a wider area of function and influence than in Western medicine. Each viscus has distinct responsibilities for maintaining the physical and psychological health of the individual. When thinking about the internal viscera according to Chinese medicine, it is more accurate to view them as spheres of influence or a network that spreads throughout the body, rather than as a distinct and separate physical organ as described by Western science. This is why the famous German sinologist, Manfred Porkert, refers to them as orbs rather than as organs. In Chinese medicine, the relationship between the various viscera and other parts of the body is made possible by the channel and network vessel system which we will discuss below.

In Chinese medicine, there are five main viscera which are relatively yin and six main bowels which are relatively yang. The five yin viscera are the heart, lungs, liver, spleen, and kidneys. The six yang bowels are the stomach, small intestine, large intestine, gallbladder, urinary bladder, and a system that Chinese medicine refers to as the triple burner. All the functions of the entire body are subsumed or described under these eleven organs or spheres of influence. Thus Chinese medicine as a system does not have a pancreas, a pituitary gland, or the ovaries. Nonetheless, all the functions of these Western organs are described under the Chinese medical system of the five viscera and six bowels.

Within this system, the five viscera are the most important. These are the organs that Chinese medicine says are responsible for the creation and transformation of qi and blood and the storage of essence. For instance, the kidneys are responsible for the excretion of urine but are also responsible for hearing, the strength of the bones, sex, reproduction, maturation and growth, the lower and upper back, and the lower legs in general and the knees in particular.

Visceral Correspondences

Organ	Tissue	Sense	Spirit	Emotion
Kidneys	bones/head hair	hearing	will	fear
Liver	sinews	sight	ethereal soul	anger
Spleen	flesh	taste	thought	thinking/worry
Lungs	skin/body hair	smell	corporeal soul	grief/sadness
Heart	blood vessels	speech	spirit	joy/fright

This points out that the Chinese viscera may have the same name and even some overlapping functions but yet are quite different from the organs of modern Western medicine. Each of the five Chinese medical viscera also has a corresponding tissue, sense, spirit, and emotion related to it. These are outlined in the table above.

In addition, each Chinese medical viscus or bowel possesses both a yin and a yang aspect. The yin aspect of a viscus or bowel refers to its substantial nature or tangible form. Further, an organ's yin is responsible for the nurturing, cooling, and moistening of that viscus or bowel. The yang aspect of the viscus or bowel represents its functional activities or what it does. An organ's yang aspect is also warming. These two aspects, yin and yang, form and function, cooling and heating, when balanced create good health. However, if either yin or yang becomes too strong or too weak, the result will be disease.

The kidneys

In Chinese medicine, the kidneys are considered to be the foundation of our life. Because the developing fetus looks like a large kidney and because the kidneys are the main viscus for the

15

storage of inherited essence, the kidneys are referred to as the prenatal root. Thus keeping the kidney qi strong and kidney yin and yang in relative balance is considered essential to good health and longevity. The basic Chinese medical statements of fact about the kidneys are:

1. The kidneys are considered responsible for human reproduction, development, and maturation.
These are the same functions we used when describing the essence. This is because the essence is stored in the kidneys. Health problems related to reproduction, development, and maturation are considered to be problems of the kidney essence. Excessive sexual activity, drug use, or simple prolonged over-exhaustion can all damage and consume kidney essence. Kidney essence is also consumed by the simple act of aging.

2. The kidneys are the foundation of water metabolism.
The kidneys work in coordination with the lungs and spleen to insure that water is spread properly throughout the body and that excess water is excreted as urination. Therefore, problems such as edema, excessive dryness, or excessive day or nighttime urination can indicate a weakness of kidney function.

3. The kidneys are responsible for hearing since the kidneys open through the portals of the ears.
Therefore, auditory problems such as diminished hearing and ringing in the ears can be due to kidney weakness.

4. The kidneys rule the grasping of qi.
This means that one of the functions of the kidney qi is to pull down or absorb the breath from the lungs and root it in the lower abdomen. Certain types of asthma and chronic cough are the result of a weakness in this kidney function.

5. The kidneys rule the bones and marrow.

This means that problems of the bones, such as osteoporosis, degenerative disc disease, and weak legs and knees, can all reflect a kidney problem.

6. Kidney yin and yang are the foundation for the yin and yang of all the other organs and bowels and body tissues of the entire body.

This is another way of saying that the kidneys are the foundation of our life. If either kidney yin or yang is insufficient, eventually the yin or yang of the other organs will also become insufficient. The clinical implications of this will become more clear when we present diabetic lower back pain case histories.

7. The kidneys store the will.

If kidney qi is insufficient, this aspect of our human nature can be weakened. Conversely, pushing ourselves to extremes, such as long distance running or cycling, can eventually exhaust our kidneys.

8. Fear is the emotion associated with the kidneys.

This means that fear can manifest when the kidney qi is insufficient. Vice versa, constant or excessive fear can damage the kidneys and make them weak.

9. The low back is the mansion of the kidneys.

This means that, of all the areas of the body, the low back is the most closely related to the health of the kidneys. If the kidneys are weak, then there may be low back pain. It is because of this and the fact that the kidneys are associated with the bones that the kidneys are the first and most important viscus in terms of the health and well-being of the low back according to Chinese medicine.

The liver

In Chinese medicine, the liver is associated with one's emotional state, with digestion, and with menstruation in women. The basic Chinese medical statements of facts concerning the liver include:

1. The liver controls coursing and discharge.

Coursing and discharge refer to the uninhibited spreading of qi to every part of the body. If the liver is not able to maintain the free and smooth flow of qi throughout the body, multiple physical and emotional symptoms can develop. This function of the liver is most easily damaged by emotional causes and, in particular, by anger and frustration. For example, if the liver is stressed due to pent-up anger, the flow of liver qi can become depressed or stagnate.

Liver qi stagnation can cause a wide range of health problems, including PMS, chronic digestive disturbance, depression, and insomnia. Therefore, it is essential to keep our liver qi flowing freely.

2. The liver stores the blood.

This means that the liver regulates the amount of blood in circulation. In particular, when the body is at rest, the blood in the extremities returns to the liver. As an extension of this, it is said in Chinese medicine that the liver is yin in form but yang in function. Thus the liver requires sufficient blood to keep it and its associated tissues moist and supple, cool and relaxed.

3. The liver controls the sinews.

The sinews refer mainly to the tendons and ligaments in the body. Proper function of the tendons and ligaments depends upon the nourishment of liver blood to keep them moist and supple.

4. The liver opens into the portals of the eyes.

The eyes are the specific sense organ corresponding to the liver. Therefore, many eye problems are related to the liver in Chinese medicine.

5. The emotion associated with the liver is anger.
Anger is the emotion that typically arises when the liver is diseased and especially when its qi does not flow freely. Conversely, anger damages the liver. Thus the emotions related to the stagnation of qi in the liver are frustration, anger, and rage.

The heart

Although the heart is the emperor of the body-mind according to Chinese medicine, it does not play as large a role in the creation and treatment of disease as one might think. Rather than the emperor initiating the cause of disease, in Chinese medicine, mostly enduring disease eventually affects the heart. Especially in terms of diabetes, disturbances of the heart tend to be secondary rather than primary. By this I mean that first some other viscus or bowel becomes diseased and then the heart feels the negative effect. The basic statements of fact about the heart in Chinese medicine are:

1. The heart governs the blood.
This means that it is the heart qi which "stirs" or moves the blood within its vessels. This is roughly analogous to the heart's pumping the blood in Western medicine. The pulsation of the blood through the arteries due to the contraction of the heart is referred to as the "stirring of the pulse." In fact, the Chinese word for pulse and vessel is the same. So this could also be translated as the "stirring of the vessels."

2. The heart stores the spirit.
The spirit refers to the mind in Chinese medicine. Therefore, this statement underscores that mental function, mental clarity, and mental equilibrium are all associated with the heart. If the heart does not receive enough qi or blood or if the heart is disturbed by something, the spirit may become restless and this may produce symptoms of mental-emotional unrest, heart palpitations, insomnia, profuse dreams, etc.

3. The heart governs the vessels.
This statement is very close to number one above. The vessels refer to the blood vessels and also to the pulse.

4. The heart governs speech.
If heart function becomes abnormal, this may be reflected in various speech problems and especially in raving and delirious speech, muttering to oneself, and speaking incoherently.

5. The heart opens into the portal of the tongue.
Because the heart has a special relationship with the tip of the tongue, heart problems may manifest as sores on the tip of the tongue.

6. Joy is the emotion associated with the heart.
The word joy has been interpreted by both Chinese and Westerners in different ways. On the one hand, joy can mean over-excitation, in which case excessive joy can cause problems with the Chinese medical functions of the heart in terms of governing the blood and storing the spirit. On the other hand, joy may be seen as an antidote to the other six emotions of Chinese medicine. From this point of view, joy causes the flow of qi (and therefore blood) to relax and become more moderate and harmonious. If some other emotion causes the qi to become bound or move chaotically, then joy can make it relax and flow normally and smoothly.

The spleen

The spleen is less important in Western medicine than it is in Chinese medicine. Since at least the Yuan dynasty (1280-1368 CE), the spleen has been one of the two most important viscera of Chinese medicine (the other being the kidneys). In Chinese medicine, the spleen plays a pivotal role in the creation of qi and blood and in the circulation and transformation of body fluids. Therefore, when it comes to the spleen, it is especially important not to think of this Chinese viscus in the same way as the

Western spleen. The main statements of fact concerning the spleen in Chinese medicine are:

1. The spleen governs movement and transformation.
This refers to the movement and transformation of foods and liquids through the digestive system. In this case, movement and transformation may be paraphrased as digestion. However, secondarily, movement and transformation also refer to the movement and transformation of body fluids through the body. It is the spleen qi which is largely responsible for controlling liquid metabolism in the body.

2. The spleen restrains the blood.
As mentioned above, one of the five functions of the qi is to restrain the fluids of the body, including the blood, within their proper channels and reservoirs. If the spleen qi is healthy and abundant, then the blood is held within its vessels properly. However, if the spleen qi becomes weak and insufficient, then the blood may flow outside its channels and vessels resulting in various types of pathological bleeding. This includes various types of pathological bleeding associated with the menstrual cycle.

3. The spleen stores the constructive.
The constructive is one of the types of qi in the body. Specifically, it is the qi responsible for nourishing and constructing the body and its tissues. This constructive qi is closely associated with the process of digestion and the creation of qi and blood out of food and liquids. If the spleen fails to store or runs out of constructive qi, then the person becomes hungry on the one hand, and eventually becomes fatigued on the other.

4. The spleen governs the muscles and flesh.
This statement is closely allied to the previous one. It is the constructive qi which constructs or nourishes the muscles and flesh. If there is sufficient spleen qi producing sufficient constructive qi, then the person's body is well-fleshed and rounded. In addition, their muscles are normally strong.

Conversely, if the spleen becomes weak, this may lead to emaciation and/or lack of strength.

5. The spleen governs the four limbs.
This means that the strength and function of the four limbs is closely associated with the spleen. If the spleen is healthy and strong, then there is sufficient strength in the four limbs and warmth in the four extremities. If the spleen becomes weak and insufficient, then there may be lack of strength in the four limbs, lack of warmth in the extremities, or even tingling and numbness in the extremities.

6. The spleen opens into the portal of the mouth.
Just as the ears are the portals of the kidneys, the eyes are the portal of the liver, the tongue is the portal of the heart, and the mouth is the portal of the spleen. Therefore, spleen disease often manifests as mouth or canker sores or bleeding from the gums.

7. Thought is the "emotion" associated with the spleen.
In the West, we do not usually think of thought as an emotion *per se*. Be that as it may, in Chinese medicine it is classified along with anger, joy, fear, grief, and melancholy. In particular, thinking, or perhaps I should say over-thinking, causes the spleen qi to bind. This means that the spleen qi does not flow harmoniously and this typically manifests as loss of appetite, abdominal bloating after meals, and indigestion.

8. The spleen is the source of engenderment and transformation.
Engenderment and transformation refer to the creation or production of the qi and blood out of the food and drink we take in each day. If the spleen receives adequate food and drink and then properly transforms that food and drink, it engenders or creates the qi and blood. Although the kidneys and lungs also participate in the creation of the qi, while the kidneys and heart also participate in the creation of the blood, the spleen is the pivotal viscus in both processes, and spleen qi weakness and

insufficiency is a leading cause of qi and blood insufficiency and weakness.

The lungs

The lungs are not one of the main Chinese viscera in the cause of diabetes. However, like the heart, the lungs often bear the brunt of disease processes initiated in other viscera and bowels. As in Western medicine, the lungs are often subject to externally invading pathogens resulting in respiratory tract diseases. However, the lungs sphere of influence also includes the skin and fluid metabolism. The main statements of fact regarding the lungs in Chinese medicine are:

1. The lungs govern the qi.
Specifically, the lungs govern the downward spread and circulation of the qi. It is the lung qi which moves all the rest of the qi in the body out to the edges and from the top of the body downward. Thus the lung qi is something like a sprinkler spraying out qi. As an extension of this, this downward qi then makes sure body fluids are moved throughout the body and eventually down to the kidneys and bladder and, eventually, out of the body.

2. The lungs govern the skin and hair.
The skin and body hair correspond with the lungs. If the lungs become diseased, this often manifests as skin problems.

3. The lungs govern the voice.
If there is sufficient lung qi, the voice is strong and clear. If there is insufficient lung qi, then the voice is weak and the person tries not to speak as a way of conserving their energy.

4. The lungs govern the free flow and regulation of the water passageways.
This statement emphasizes the role of lung qi in moving body fluids outward and downward throughout the body, ultimately to arrive at the urinary bladder. If the lung qi fails to maintain the

free flow and regulation of the water passageways, then fluids will collect and transform into dampness, thus producing water swelling or edema.

5. The lungs govern the defensive exterior.

We say above that the qi defends the body against invasion by external pathogens. In Chinese medicine, the exterior-most layer of the body is the area where the defensive qi circulates and the place where this defense, therefore, takes place. In particular, it is the lungs which govern this defensive qi. If the lungs function normally and there is sufficient defensive qi, then the body cannot be invaded by external pathogens. If the lungs are weak and the defensive qi is insufficient, then external pathogens may easily invade the exterior of the body, causing complaints such as colds, flus, and allergies.

6. The lungs are the florid canopy.

This means that the lungs are like a tent spreading over the top of all the other viscera and bowels. On the one hand, they are the first viscus to be assaulted by external pathogens invading the body from the top. On the other, any pathogenic qi moving upward in the body eventually may accumulate in and affect the lungs.

7. The lungs are the delicate viscus.

Because the lungs are the most delicate of all the viscera and bowels, they are the most easily invaded by external pathogens. This is the Chinese explanation for the prevalence of colds and flus in comparison to other types of diseases.

8. The lungs form snivel.

This means that snivel or nasal mucus has to do, at least in part, with lung function. If the lungs are functioning correctly, there should not be any runny nose or nasal congestion.

9. The lungs open into the portal of the nose.
This statement is similar to the one above. However, it approaches the issue from a slightly different perspective. The implication of this statement is that diseases having to do with the nose and its function are often associated with the Chinese medical idea of the lungs.

Each yin viscus is paired with a yang bowel in a yin-yang or interior-exterior relationship. The kidneys are paired with the urinary bladder, the liver is paired with the gallbladder, the heart is paired with the small intestine, the spleen is paired with the stomach, and the lungs are paired with the large intestine. The yin viscus is relatively more interior and the yang bowel is relatively more exterior. In the case of the urinary bladder, gallbladder, and stomach, these bowels receive their qi from their paired viscus and function very much as an extension of that viscus. The relationship between the other two viscera and bowels is not as close.

The gallbladder

The main statements of fact concerning the gallbladder in terms of diabetes in Chinese medicine are:

1. The gallbladder governs decision.
In Chinese medicine, the liver is likened to a general who plans strategy for the body, while the gallbladder is likened to a judge. According to this point of view, if a person lacks gallbladder qi, they will have trouble making decisions. In addition, they will be timid. While courage in the West is associated with the heart (*coeur* = courage), bravery in the East is associated with the gallbladder. Actually, this is also an old Western idea as well. When someone is very forward and brazen, we say that "They have gall." Conversely, if someone is excessively timid, this may be due to gallbladder qi vacuity or insufficiency. In Chinese medicine, this is called "gallbladder timidity."

25

2. The liver and gallbladder have the same palace.
This statement underscores the particularly close relationship between the liver and gallbladder.

3. If there is qi because of a robust gallbladder, evils are not able to enter.
These two statements are very close to statements in Chinese medicine about the heart saying that the heart is the sovereign of the body and that if spirit abides (in the heart), then evils cannot enter. Both these statements elevate the gallbladder to a place of importance in the body it does not hold in Western medicine and link the gallbladder in a way to the heart and its spirit.

The stomach

There are a number of important statements of fact concerning the stomach in Chinese medicine due to the stomach's pivotal role in digestion and, therefore, in the creation of qi and blood. Below we will only discuss those statements which we will use later in our discussion of the disease causes and disease mechanisms of diabetes in Chinese medicine.

1. The stomach governs intake.
This means that the stomach is the first to receive foods and drinks ingested into the body.

2. The stomach governs downbearing of the turbid.
The process of digestion in Chinese medicine is likened to the process of fermentation and then distillation. The stomach is the fermentation tun wherein foods and liquids are "rottened and ripened." This rottening and ripening allows for the separation of clear and turbid parts of the digestate. The spleen sends the clear parts upward to the lungs and heart to become the qi and blood respectively. The stomach's job is to send the turbid part down to be excreted as waste from the large intestine and bladder.

3. Stomach heat may exploit the heart.
If, for any reason, abnormal or pathological heat collects in the stomach, because heat is yang and has an innate tendency to move upward and outward, and because the heart is located above the stomach in Chinese medicine, heat in the stomach may exploit or harass the heart above.

The triple burner

Above I mentioned that there are five viscera and six bowels. The sixth bowel is called the triple burner. It is said in Chinese that, "The triple burner has a function but no form." The name triple burner refers to the three main areas of the torso. The upper burner is the chest. The middle burner is the space from the bottom of the rib-cage to the level of the navel. The lower burner is the lower abdomen below the navel. These three spaces are called burners because all of the functions and transformations of the viscera and bowels which they contain are "warm" transformations similar to food cooking in a pot on a stove or similar to an alchemical transformation in a furnace. In fact, the triple burner is nothing other than a generalized concept of how the other viscera and bowels function together as an organic unit in terms of the digestion of foods and liquids and the circulation and transformation of body fluids.

The Channels & Network Vessels

Each viscus and bowel has a corresponding channel with which it is connected. In Chinese medicine, the inside of the body is made up of the viscera and bowels. The outside of the body is composed of the sinews and bones, muscles and flesh, and skin and hair. It is the channels and network vessels (*i.e.,* smaller connecting vessels) which connect the inside and the outside of the body. It is through these channels and network vessels that the viscera and bowels connect with their corresponding body tissues.

The channels and network vessel system is a unique feature of traditional Chinese medicine. These channels and vessels are different from the circulatory, nervous, or lymphatic systems. The earliest reference to these channels and vessels is in *Nei Jing (Inner Classic)*, a text written around the 2nd or 3rd century BCE.

The channels and vessels perform two basic functions. They are the pathways by which the qi and blood circulate through the body and between the organs and tissues. Additionally, as mentioned above, the channels connect the viscera and bowels internally with the exterior part of the body. This channel and vessel system functions in the body much like the world information communication network. The channels allow the various parts of our body to cooperate and interact to maintain our lives.

This channel and network vessel system is complex. There are 12 primary channels, 6 yin and 6 yang, each with a specific pathway through the external body and connected with an internal organ (see diagrams below). There are also extraordinary vessels, sinew channels, channel divergences, main network vessels, and ultimately countless finer and finer network vessels permeating the entire body. All of these form a closed loop or circuit similar to but distinct from the Western circulatory system.

Acupuncture points are places located on the major channels where there is a special concentration of qi and blood. Because of the relatively more qi and blood accumulated at these places, the sites act as switches which can potentially control the flow of qi and blood in the channel on which the point is located. By stimulating these points in any of a number of different ways, one can speed up or slow down, make more or reduce, warm or cool down the qi and blood flowing in the channels and vessels. The main ways of stimulating these points and thus adjusting the flow of qi and blood in the channels and vessels is to needle them and to heat them by moxibustion. Moxibustion refers to the burning of Chinese mugwort either on or over an acupuncture point. Other commonly used ways of stimulating these points and thus adjusting the qi and blood flowing through the channels and vessels are massage, cupping, the application of magnets, and the application of various herbal medicinals. If the channels and vessels are the pathways over which the qi and blood flow, then the acupuncture points are the places where this flow can be adjusted.

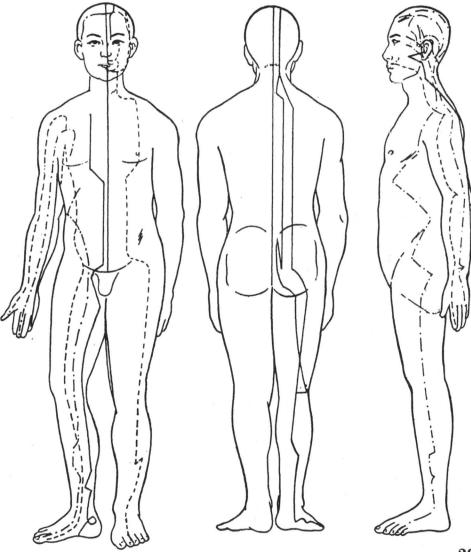

The Chinese Medical View of Digestion

Because faulty diet is the root cause of diabetes in Chinese medicine, before we can understand its disease mechanisms we must first have some idea about how Chinese medicine describes digestion. After all, faulty diet first and foremost affects the organs of digestion.

The spleen & stomach

According to Chinese medical theory, the spleen and stomach are the main organs of digestion. These two have what is called an interior-exterior relationship. That means they are a yin-yang pair something like a husband and wife team. The spleen is yin and located more interior, while the stomach is yang and located more exterior. When we eat, food and liquids go directly to the stomach where they are initially broken down or decomposed. This is called "rottening and ripening" in Chinese, and the stomach is likened to a fermentation tun or vat. Then the spleen transforms and separates the clear and turbid parts of this digestive mash. The clear or pure parts of the digestate, also called the finest essence of food and liquids, is transformed into the qi and blood and sent upward to the heart and lungs for distribution to the rest of the body. Because the spleen is the root of qi and blood production, it's health and proper function are vital to the health and proper function of the entire rest of the body.

When we are born, the spleen and stomach are inherently immature and weak. It takes until we are six or seven years old for the spleen and stomach to mature and become strongly and efficiently functioning. According to the *Nei Jing (Inner Classic)*, the stomach and intestines and, therefore, the spleen, begin to become weak and inefficient due to aging at around 35 years of age. What this means is that, at around 35 years of age, due to a lifetime of diseases, injuries, and dietary insults, spleen and stomach function begin to decline, and with this decline, comes an accompanying decline in the spleen's production of qi and blood.

What happens in the intestines?

In Chinese medicine, the stomach and intestines are typically talked about as a unit. Therefore, intestinal function is often subsumed under stomach function. When the spleen sends the finest essence or the clear part of the digestate upwards to become the qi and blood, the stomach sends the turbid residue downwards. This is referred to as the upbearing of the clear and the downbearing of the turbid. The small intestine sends the liquid part of this residue to the bladder for excretion as urine, while the large intestine excretes the solid part of this residue as feces.

The role of the liver in digestion

In Chinese medicine, the liver is not considered one of the digestive organs *per se*. However, the liver governs coursing and discharging. This refers to the free flow of the qi. Now the upbearing of the clear and the downbearing of the turbid by the stomach (and, by extension, the intestines) is referred to as the qi mechanism, and this qi mechanism can only function properly if the qi is freely flowing. Therefore, if, for any reason, the liver's coursing and discharging is hindered or damaged, this may inhibit the free flow of the qi mechanism. And if the qi mechanism is inhibited, this means that the digestive functions of the spleen and stomach may be impaired. What is the main cause of the liver's losing its control over the coursing and discharging of the qi? In Chinese, that is literally referred to as "unfulfilled desires," but we can read this as stress, frustration, and emotional upset.

The role of the kidneys in digestion

Likewise, in Chinese medicine, the kidneys are not considered digestive organs. Nevertheless, they do play an indirect role in the digestive process. The kidneys control the lifegate fire. This is another name for kidney yang or kidney fire. Kidney yang is like the pilot light of the body which "warms and steams" all the other viscera and bowels allowing them to do their duty. All physiological transformations in the body are warm transformations according to Chinese medicine, since all transformations are a function of yang qi which is inherently warm. In particular, the spleen cannot carry out its functions of engendering and transforming the qi and blood without support from kidney yang below. Therefore, if spleen qi becomes vacuous (meaning insufficient) and weak, this may eventually cause the kidney yang to likewise become weak and insufficient. Vice versa, if kidney yang were, for any reason, to become vacuous and weak, this would also result in the spleen becoming vacuous and weak.

In addition, the spleen, stomach, and kidneys are intimately connected in terms of fluid metabolism. Fluids in the body originate in the stomach. The pure part of fluids from the digestate are moved and transformed by the spleen, which means that the spleen qi moves them up to the lungs to be spread throughout the body by the power of lung qi which also comes from the spleen. The impure part is sent down from the stomach to the bladder (via the small intestine). The bladder qi is derived from the kidney qi. (These two are a yin-yang pair.)

Hence, there is also a close relationship between the stomach and the kidneys in terms of fluid metabolism. In Chinese medicine, it is said that, "The kidneys are the bar of the stomach." This means that the kidney qi holds the bladder closed in order to store the fluids sent down to the bladder by the stomach. If the stomach is overheated and hyperfunctioning, sending too many liquids down to the bladder for excretion, eventually, the kidney qi will become exhausted. This is because it is the kidney qi which is the root of the bladder qi which must move and discharge these liquids out of the body.

The main cause of kidney weakness in clinical practice is aging, although the Chinese literature also says the kidneys can be damaged by too much sex, and certainly in modern times, the Chinese kidneys can be damaged by both "recreational" drugs, like cocaine and amphetamines, and prescription drugs, such as prednisone and other corticosteroids.

Since the spleen governs the muscles and flesh, both obesity and emaciation are primarily seen in Chinese medicine as pathological changes in the spleen. Since the spleen and stomach "open into" the mouth, changes in the taste in the mouth, such as bland, slimy, and sweet tastes or feelings, are also related to pathological changes in these two organs. Further, changes in appetite, either poor appetite or ravenous hunger, are usually indicative of disease processes affecting these two organs.

The five flavors

According to Chinese medical theory, every food has some combination of the five flavors. These five flavors are sweet, sour, bitter, acrid, and salty. The five flavors are intimately associated with the clear or pure part of food. Each of these five flavors primarily enters or gathers in one of the five yin viscera. Thus it is said that sweet gathers in the spleen, sour gathers in the liver, bitter gathers in the heart, acridity (*i.e.*, pungent, spicy flavors) gather in the lungs, and salty gathers in the kidneys. Each of these flavors feed the qi of the corresponding viscus. Therefore, we need all five of these flavors in moderate amounts in order to be healthy. However, when overeaten, each of these five flavors damages the viscus it gathers in.

Diet & health

The *Nei Jing (Inner Classic)*, the "Bible" of Chinese medicine mentioned above, discusses the relationship of humans to the cosmos and correct human behavior to maintain good health. Among its many precepts is advice on good eating habits. When this correct behavior in eating is followed, good health is the result. The *Nei Jing* says:

> One should be mindful of what one consumes to insure proper growth, reproduction, and development of bones, sinews, channels, and network vessels. This will help promote the smooth flow of qi and blood, enabling one to live to a ripe age.

Here the *Nei Jing* directly relates healthy living and even longevity to good everyday eating habits. This ancient classic goes on to say that any of the flavors when consumed in excess can cause disease. Thus moderation in eating habits is the key to health, for any excess of the five flavors brings about imbalance.

The Chinese Mechanisms of Diabetes

In ancient China, what we now call diabetes was traditionally called *xiao ke*. *Xiao ke* literally means "flowing away and thirst." This refers to the great thirst of the patient and the flowing away of larger than normal amounts of fluids via urination.[1] *Xiao ke* was recognized as a specific disease as early as the second century BCE when it was described as being the result of long-term consumption of fatty, rich, and sweet foods. The term diabetes mellitus, as it is used in modern Western medicine, is actually a mix of Greek and Latin terms. Diabetes in Greek describes the process of "flowing through," referring to the excessive urination which even a great thirst cannot replace. In this sense, the Greek term is surprisingly similar to the Chinese *xiao ke* in describing this pathological process. The term mellitus, derived from the Latin word *mel* or honey, refers to the sweet taste and smell of the patient's urine. In modern Chinese medical texts, diabetes is called *tang niao bing* or "sugar urine disease." This nomenclature needs no explanation, for it is a literal description of this disorder, emphasizing not only the loss of fluids through urination, but also the excessive sweetness of that urine.

---

[1] Some translators render this term as "wasting and thirsting," thus emphasizing the weight loss and thirst which characterize this disease. One of the beauties of the Chinese language is that a single word or term can mean several things at the same time.

Now that we've gone over basic Chinese medical theory and discussed digestion from the Chinese point of view, we can look at the specific causes and mechanisms of diabetes identified in Chinese medicine. As stated above, as early as the second century BCE, Chinese doctors have known that diabetes is due to "overeating fatty, rich, and sweet foods." In an article titled "Overeating Sugars & Sweets [Causes] Detriment & Damage to the Five Viscera," Bu Lu-nuo and Bu Lu-ke, two contemporary Chinese doctors, discuss the relationship between overeating sugar and sweets and hypoglycemia and diabetes.[2] Bu and Bu say that overeating sweet flavored foods do two things. First they damage the spleen and, secondly, this disease then reaches the five viscera.

Bu and Bu begin by quoting the *Su Wen (Simple Questions)*, the first book of the *Nei Jing (Inner Classic)*:

> The five flavors enter the stomach, each gathering where there is a liking for it... Sweet first enters the spleen...

Sweetness can boost or strengthen the spleen, but in large amounts, it can also congest the center. Overeating sweet foods and drinks is, therefore, also able to damage the spleen. Because the spleen is no longer able to move and transport body fluids properly, these gather and accumulate and transform into dampness and phlegm which then go on to obstruct and stagnate the flow of the qi. Because the spleen is the root of qi and blood engenderment and transformation, both the qi and blood become vacuous and debilitated. Spleen vacuity due to damage by overeating sweets manifests as abdominal distention after meals, fatigue, lack of strength, somnolence, bodily obesity, and possible lower limb swelling and edema.

---

[2] Bu Lu-nuo & Bu Lu-ke, *Jiang Xi Zhong Yi Yao (Jiangxi Chinese Medicine & Medicinals)*, #1, 1995, p. 58

Bu and Bu also astutely and correctly recognize that many people who are addicted to sweets also suffer from psycho-emotional tension. This relationship between a craving for sweets and emotional tension is due to two separate but interlinked disease mechanisms. First, if the liver becomes depressed due to stress and frustration, it typically "counterflows" onto or attacks the spleen which then becomes vacuous and weak. The sweet flavor boosts the spleen qi. So it is only natural that, when the spleen is vacuous and weak, it craves the sweet flavor. Unfortunately for us, overeating sweets or eating intensely sweet foods (as opposed to the natural sweetness in most grains, vegetables, and meats) further damages the spleen.

Secondly, it is said in Chinese medicine that the sweet flavor relaxes tension: "[When there is] tension, eating sweet things automatically remedies this." This means that people under stress automatically crave sugars and sweets as a way to not only boost their qi or energy but also as a way to relax that tension.

Bu and Bu state that most people in the early stages of hypoglycemia exhibit this situation. Because they have eaten a large amount of sugar, their spleen function has suffered detriment and damage. This gives rise to a liver-spleen disharmony with the patient exhibiting emotional depression combined with a short-tempered, agitated disposition. If the spleen becomes weak, dampness and phlegm obstruct internally, manifesting as fright and fear and insomnia. If the spleen becomes weak, then the qi and blood become vacuous and insufficient. Hence the liver loses its nourishment, along with the tissues corresponding to the liver, *i.e.*, the sinews, the nails, the genitalia, and the eyes. The heart loses its nourishment and thus the spirit treasured by the heart becomes agitated. This may result in insomnia, nervous agitation, anxiety, and heart palpitations. If the spleen becomes weak, then the lungs must also become weak, since the lungs get their qi directly from the spleen. Likewise, because of the reciprocal relationship between the spleen and the kidneys, if the spleen becomes weak, the kidneys must also eventually suffer detriment and damage. Thus all five viscera may become affected if emotional tension causes the liver to become depressed and overeating sweets damages the spleen.

What 'Bu and Bu do not discuss is the tendency for the stomach to become overheated in this process. When the liver becomes depressed, it also tends to become overheated. This depressive or transformative heat is often transferred to or affects the stomach. In addition, the stomach may also become overheated due to overeating in general and overeating certain specific types of foods in particular. These include greasy, fatty, and/or fried foods; spicy, hot, peppery foods; and, paradoxically, chilled, frozen foods.

Pathological heat in the stomach will eventually do two things. First, it will tend to flare upward, thus affecting the lungs and heart above, as well as the sensory organs in the upper extremity, the head. Secondly, if it continues and endures, it will eventually consume and damage yin. This means that pathological heat in the stomach may be transferred to the lungs and heart and may result in yin vacuity of the heart, lungs, spleen, stomach, liver, and kidneys. In addition, either a yin and blood vacuity or internal heat may give rise to internally stirring of liver wind.

Bu and Bu also do not say anything about blood stasis. If the liver qi is depressed and bound and the spleen qi is vacuous and weak, then the blood must eventually become static. This is because:

> The qi moves the blood. If the qi moves, the blood moves. If the qi stops, the blood stops.

Therefore, enduring qi stagnation must eventually lead to blood stasis, and this is even more likely if the spleen qi has become weak. It is the spleen qi which becomes the heart qi which moves or pushes the blood, while it is the spleen which manufactures the blood which nourishes the blood vessels. If the blood vessels lose their nourishment, then they cannot play their role in promoting the flow of blood. Further, if phlegm and dampness are obstructing the free flow of qi and blood, one has a perfect recipe for blood stasis.

The seven basic disease mechanisms of diabetes

Thus there are seven basic causes and mechanisms of diabetes in Chinese medicine. Each of these causes leads to imbalances in digestion and disrupts the upbearing and downbearing functions of the spleen and stomach. When this happens, the yin and yang of the body are not nourished, yin fluids become depleted, and yin is consumed and fails to control yang, resulting in yang counterflowing upward and outward. Also, since yin and yang are rooted in each other, yin vacuity may eventually result in yang vacuity.

1. Stomach heat exuberance

Stomach heat is a very common interior heat pattern seen in clinic. It may occur when evil (*i.e.*, pathogenic or pathological) heat enters the stomach from the outside as in a case of the flu. However, stomach heat is most often the result of overeating rich, hot, greasy, fried, fatty, and spicy foods and overindulgence in alcohol. Likewise, although most sugars are categorized as cool, excessive consumption of sugars and sweets can also indirectly or eventually result in stomach heat. Another cause of stomach heat is overeating or overdrinking chilled, iced frozen foods. When something ice cold lands in the stomach, the stomach has to go into high gear or overdrive to "cook" this food into 100°F soup. If this happens over and over again, the stomach may become "stuck in overdrive" or permanently overheated.

There are two other common causes of stomach heat. In Chinese medicine, the stomach is closely related to both the liver and the lungs. If the liver becomes depressed and the qi becomes stagnant due to emotional stress, anger, and frustration, this stuck qi may accumulate like hot air in an over-pressurized tire. Because qi is

41

yang, an accumulation of qi will transform into heat. Thus, if liver
depression transforms into depressive or transformative heat,
this heat may also be transferred to the stomach.

Secondly, if the lungs become hot and dry due to smoking tobacco,
this may eventually result in simultaneous stomach heat. Tobacco
smoke is hot, acrid, and drying according to Chinese medicine. Its
smoking results in the lungs becoming overheated and their yin
fluids suffering damage. Lung yin fluids come from stomach
fluids. Thus a lung yin vacuity or insufficiency may eventually
result in a stomach fluid dryness and insufficiency. Since yin
controls and holds yang in check, stomach yin vacuity is typically
complicated by stomach yang hyperactivity or what is more
commonly referred to as stomach heat.

If there is pathological heat in the stomach, this heat will waft
upwards to affect the heart and lungs. It will also damage and
consume yin fluids throughout the body. Just as a lung yin
vacuity may eventually cause a stomach yin vacuity, a stomach
yin vacuity may eventually cause a yin vacuity of the heart,
lungs, liver, spleen, and/or kidneys. Further, the stomach qi
should downbear and descend, but heat is a yang evil. This means
heat inherently tends to rise. Therefore, heat in the stomach is
often associated with the stomach's loss of downbearing or what
is technically referred to as the stomach's loss of harmony.

2. Liver depression qi stagnation
As we have seen above, the liver governs the coursing and
discharge of all the qi in the body. This means that the liver
ensures that the flow of qi is smooth and freely flowing. If a
person's desires are unfulfilled, this is saying that the flow of
their qi cannot "spread freely." This frustration in turn affects the
liver's coursing and discharging of the qi. Proportional to the
frustration, the liver's coursing and discharging of the qi will
become depressed and the qi flow stagnant. This is called liver
depression qi stagnation. It is mostly due to stress and frustration
or the non-attainment of one's desires. Because no adult can
fulfill all one's desires at the very moment we desire them, most

adults suffer from some element of liver depression qi stagnation, and, typically, the more stress and frustration, the more liver depression and qi stagnation.

In actual fact, liver depression qi stagnation due to emotional stress and frustration does not cause diabetes all by itself. However, if the liver becomes depressed, this typically leads to the spleen becoming vacuous and weak. This is because the liver "controls" the spleen according to an ancient Chinese theory called five phase theory. Based on this theory, the spleen is usually the first viscus to subsequently become diseased after the liver becomes depressed. If the spleen becomes vacuous and weak, it will not engender and transform the qi and blood properly, and this then may lead to malnourishment of the rest of the body.

There is a theory in Chinese medicine called the theory of similar transformation which we've alluded to above. Because the body's living qi is yang and, therefore, warm in nature, if anything causes this qi to accumulate and not flow freely, it may cause such depressed and stagnant yang qi to transform into pathological heat. Therefore, it is said in Chinese medicine that enduring liver depression due to emotional stress and frustration may transform into heat or fire. This is called transformative or depressive heat. This transformation may also take place in a shorter period of time if frustration and stress give way to outright anger. It is said in Chinese medicine that, "Any of the seven emotions may transform into fire if extreme."

Fire is by nature yang and, therefore, tends to move upward and outward in the body, drafting along with it the body's host yang qi. In addition, this fire tends to collect in the upper part of the body and in the lungs and heart.

This tendency of depressive heat due to stress and frustration or anger and emotional upset to rise up and accumulate in the heart or lungs can be aggravated by eating hot, acrid, peppery foods. This includes chilis and peppers, but also greasy, fried, fatty foods, and alcohol, sweets, and coffee. Overeating any of these can give rise to stomach heat which then mutually aggravates and engenders liver heat.

Because heat or fire is yang, it not only moves upward and outward in the body but also evaporates and consumes blood and yin. As we age, because yin is already half consumed, there is a tendency for depression to transform into heat even more easily. If depressive heat endures for a long time in the body, it will consume and damage the yin of the liver and kidneys. This then leads to kidney essence depletion and vacuity. The liver loses its ability to moisten and nourish the sinews and is not able to restrain yang. If yang moves frenetically or chaotically, this is referred to as "internal stirring of liver wind."

3. Yin vacuity, fire effulgence
When yin becomes truly vacuous and insufficient, yang may become hyperactive. If yang becomes very hyperactive, it is called internal fire. Since yin is primarily associated with the kidneys and hyperactive yang is primarily associated with the liver, this is also referred to as kidney yin vacuity with ascendant hyperactivity of liver yang or liver yang harassing and stirring above. Such a kidney yin vacuity may be due to constitutional insufficiency, meaning that the person was simply not born with much yin to begin with. People with very thin bodies tend to suffer from constitutional yin vacuity. Such yin vacuity can be due to aging as we have already seen. Such yin vacuity may also be due to long-term or severe disease and especially a febrile or feverish disease. In that case, the pathological heat associated with the disease consumes and wastes the body's yin blood. Tuberculosis, or what is still called vacuity consumption in Chinese medicine, is a good example of this mechanism.

It is also possible for yin vacuity to be due to simply too much stirring or activity. In Chinese, the word _dong_ means to stir. In the Jin-Yuan dynasties, Zhu Dan-xi, the last of the four great doctors of that era, said that, in human beings in general, "Yang tends to be superabundant, while yin is typically insufficient" and that any activity may cause stirring of yang and further consumption of yin. By activity, Zhu meant any physical, mental, or emotional activity. Zhu saw all these activities as manifestations of stirring yang which consumes yin and leads to only more stirring of yang.

In particular, Zhu singled out what, in Chinese, is referred to as "bedroom taxation." Simply put, this means too much sex, and both men and women can suffer from it. Sexual desire in Chinese medicine is a preeminent manifestation of stirring yang. When we are filled with sexual desire, we say we are "hot" with desire. We are all "stirred up." We are "hot and bothered." And we need to take a cold shower to douse "the flames of our desire." All these colloquialisms point to the same truth that the Chinese have known for centuries. In Chinese medicine, sexual desire and sexual activity are both a function of kidney fire or kidney yang. If sexual desire is not fulfilled, then this fire is stirred up and then depressed. This leads to liver depression transforming into heat. If the desire is fulfilled, this leads to consumption and loss of yin. In either case, too much desire or too much sex can lead to or worsen yin vacuity with its attendant loss of control over yang.

Likewise, anything which speeds up the body or pushes the body to prolonged excessive activity may lead to yin vacuity and yang hyperactivity. Things which speed up the body are caffeinated drinks, such as coffee, and recreational drugs, such as cocaine and amphetamines (or speed). Prolonged, excessive stirring refers to prolonged, excessive emotions or prolonged excessive activity, such as too much exercise. Any of these can waste yin and stir yang hyperactively. In our modern context, this includes "sex, drugs, and rock n' roll."

If yin becomes extremely vacuous and yang fire becomes extremely hyperactive, yin and yang may come apart and fail to interact in a harmonious and healthy way. Since water is yin and the kidneys are the water viscus according to five phase theory, an ancient system of reciprocal correspondence in Chinese medicine, while fire is yang and the heart is the fire viscus, such an extreme coming apart of yin and yang is sometimes referred to as heart and kidneys not interacting.

4. Qi & yin dual vacuity

If thinking, worry, over-taxation, or fatigue are excessive, any of these may damage the spleen. Thinking is a yang activity of the spirit which consumes yin blood. If thinking is excessive, then there will be excessive consumption of yin blood. Because the spleen is the root of qi and blood engenderment and transformation, spleen qi which is vacuous and weak will fail to manufacture and send enough blood to the heart spirit. When heart yin is not sufficient, the heart loses its nourishment. The spleen qi will also fail to make the blood which will nourish the lungs resulting in lung qi and yin vacuity with vacuity heat and depletion of lung fluids. When lung qi is not sufficient, there is also insecurity of the defensive exterior.

Although Chinese medical texts tend to emphasize the negative role of over-thinking and too much work, too little exercise and faulty diet may also contribute to a qi and yin dual vacuity. While too much work or exercise overly consumes the qi and blood manufactured by the spleen, too little exercise causes the qi mechanism to become stagnant. The qi mechanism is the mechanism of upbearing the pure or clear part of the digestate and downbearing the turbid part. This upbearing and downbearing is dependent on the free and active flow of qi. When one fails to get sufficient exercise, the qi does not flow smoothly and freely, and so upbearing and downbearing and the consequent engenderment and transformation of qi and blood is also sluggish and insufficient.

In addition, eating the wrong foods may also damage the spleen, thus resulting in a heart blood vacuity. The process of digestion is a warm transformation of yang qi working on and refining yin substance. Therefore, eating too many chilled and uncooked foods and drinking iced liquids can douse the digestive fire of the spleen.[3] Likewise, eating too many sugars and sweets may also damage the spleen. This includes too many sweet and juicy fruits and fruit juices, like oranges and peaches. And finally, eating too many dairy products and fatty foods may damage the spleen, leading to spleen vacuity and consequent qi and blood vacuity.

The inability of the spleen to provide strength and nourishment to the rest of the body also affects the functions of the liver and the kidneys. If the spleen cannot produce qi and blood, then the liver, whose function it is to store the blood, will receive less and less yin blood. This means that the liver becomes vacuous and weak. In turn, the liver blood does not nourish the heart, and the heart spirit becomes restless. When the spleen can no longer produce qi and blood, it will look to the kidneys as the supplier of yin essence to make up the difference. Over time, this leaves the kidney yin and blood depleted and weak. When kidney yin becomes depleted, yang qi floats upward accompanied by vacuity heat.

Dual vacuity of qi and blood can be caused by the spleen's inability to contain the blood. In Chinese medicine, we call this the "qi not managing the blood." When this happens, the spleen qi is so weak that it cannot contain or restrain the blood in its vessels. Bleeding results along with blood vacuity. Hence there is insufficient blood to moisten and nourish the sinews and vessels. This may lead to blood vacuity alone or, over time, result also in blood stasis as we shall discuss below.

5. Yin & yang dual vacuities
In Chinese medicine, we say that yin and yang are rooted in each other. That means that yin and yang are interdependent and mutually engendering. Damage to yin affects yang, and damage

---

[3] Eating chilled and uncooked foods does different things to the spleen and stomach. In Westerners, at least, the tendency is for the stomach to become overheated while the spleen becomes cold and damp.

to yang affects yin. When the damage is great or exists over a long period of time, a yin and yang dual vacuity will result.

It is also said in Chinese medicine that, "Enduring disease reaches the kidneys." This means that any enduring disease may eventually damage and weaken the kidneys. Kidney yang is the root of the yang for the entire body, and kidney yang vacuity can cause a yang and/or qi vacuity of other viscera, namely, the spleen, lungs, and heart. In turn, vacuity of the spleen, lungs, and heart may also cause or contribute to vacuity of kidney yang. Kidney yang warms the body and the other organs and is responsible for sexual desire and performance. It also has the functions of transforming water and storing the essence. When kidney yin has suffered detriment over time, kidney yang can no longer support these functions.

Without kidney yang to warm and steam the spleen yang qi, proper digestion cannot occur. Thus, proper kidney function is essential to maintaining life. If the spleen cannot perform its functions of movement and transformation, then the processes of upbearing and downbearing, which we discussed earlier, will not proceed smoothly and efficiently. Consequently, the sinews and vessels will be deprived of moisture and nourishment, and all other functions of the body may become impaired. In addition, the spleen will not be able to transform water and warm the body, so dampness and phlegm will accumulate, the defensive exterior will weaken, and the limbs will no longer be strong.

As we discussed in chapter 3, digestion may also be impaired by improper eating habits and dietary irregularities. Overeating raw, chilled foods, overindulging in cold, icy drinks, or imbalanced vegetarian regimes may all weaken the spleen's yang qi and cause spleen qi vacuity. This in turn will affect the kidney yang as well, since the spleen must depend more and more on the kidneys to substitute for its own yang qi.

When spleen qi and kidney yang become vacuous and weak, they cannot warm lung and heart yang qi either. This results in yin cold becoming exuberant within the body, read dampness and phlegm, and qi and blood movement in the channels and vessels slows down. Qi and blood cannot nourish and moisten, and, over time, blood stasis results and water and dampness accumulate internally. This will affect the ability of the heart to govern, *i.e.*, move or pump, the blood and to house the heart spirit. The lungs will be unable to defend the exterior and to govern the qi of the body.

6. Blood stasis

The Chinese word for stasis is derived from the Chinese word for silt. Therefore, static blood is seen as a kind of dry, dead, or wrecked blood which silts up and, hence, obstructs the channels and vessels. Such blood stasis may be due to traumatic injury, long-standing liver depression qi stagnation failing to move the blood, qi vacuity failing to push the blood, cold congealing the blood, or insufficient blood to nourish the vessels and keep them open and functioning correctly. In Chinese medicine, it is a given that static blood hinders the creation of new or fresh blood. This means that blood stasis may give rise to blood vacuity and blood vacuity may give rise to blood stasis.

In cases of diabetes, blood stasis is not usually one of the disease causes listed in Chinese medical textbooks. However, most diabetics exhibit some signs and symptoms of blood stasis. This is because, as stated above, the qi moves the blood. If, for any reason, the qi is not strong enough to move the blood, if there is something hindering or obstructing the free movement of qi and blood, such as dampness and/or phlegm, or if the liver is not allowing the free movement of the qi, then blood stasis will eventually also arise. Therefore, blood stasis typically complicates most chronic and enduring diseases. Since diabetes directly affects the spleen, heart, lungs, liver, and kidneys, all the viscera which, in Chinese medicine either engender and transform the qi and blood or promote their free and uninhibited flow, it is no wonder that diabetics almost always show some signs and symptoms of blood stasis.

7. Water dampness accumulating internally and congealing into phlegm

Overindulgence in greasy, fatty, fried foods, hot, acrid, peppery foods, and alcohol, and overeating sugar and sweets as well as raw, chilled foods can all cause damage to the spleen. In that case, the spleen cannot perform its functions of movement and transformation of body fluids. Instead, these fluids will gather and collect, transforming into pathological dampness. If this dampness gathers and endures and then is further acted upon by either heat or cold, it may congeal into phlegm. Phlegm may hinder and obstruct the free flow of qi and blood. Phlegm may block any of the orifices of the body. These orifices include the eyes, ears, nose, and mouth, the urethra, and the "orifices of the heart." If the eyes, ears, nose, mouth, or urethra are blocked by phlegm, they cannot carry out their respective functions. If the orifices of the heart are "confounded" or blocked by phlegm, the heart spirit is affected. This then results in either mental-emotional restlessness and agitation, lack of consciousness, or impaired intelligence. In addition, phlegm can flow into the spaces between the skin and muscles to accumulate as adipose tissue and/or fatty tumors, such as lipomas.

As the reader can see from the above descriptions, there are a number of different causes and mechanisms for diabetes in different people. In most cases, faulty diet affecting the spleen and stomach is the main cause. However, depending on the individual, this is then complicated by aging, mental-emotional stress, too much or too little exercise, and other factors such as smoking and drug use, both so-called recreational and therapeutic.

Because there are different Chinese causes of diabetes in different people, no one treatment is right for everyone. When a particular treatment is wrong for a particular person, then either or both of two things happen. First, the treatment is ineffective. It doesn't do what it is supposed to do. And secondly, it may cause unwanted side effects. On the bright side, if one can identify their Chinese pattern of diabetes, one can immediately know what they as individuals should and should not do, eat and not eat. Further, because just the right treatment is given to the right individual, Chinese medicine heals without side effects or doctor-caused complications.

The Chinese Medical Treatment of Diabetes

The hallmark of professional Chinese medicine is what is known as "treatment based on pattern discrimination." Modern Western medicine bases its treatment on a disease diagnosis. This means that two patients diagnosed as suffering from the same disease will get the same treatment. Traditional Chinese medicine also takes the patient's disease diagnosis into account. However, the choice of treatment is not based on the disease so much as it is on what is called the patient's pattern, and it is treatment based on pattern discrimination which is what makes Chinese medicine the holistic, safe, and effective medicine it is.

In order to explain the difference between a disease and a pattern, let us take headache for example. Everyone who is diagnosed as suffering from a headache has to, by definition, have some pain in their head. In modern Western medicine and other medical systems which primarily prescribe on the basis of a disease diagnosis, one can talk about "headache medicines." However, amongst headache sufferers, one may be a man and the other a woman. One may be old and the other young. One may be fat and the other skinny. One may have pain on the right side of her head and the other may have pain on the left. In one case, the pain may be throbbing and continuous, while the other person's pain may be very sharp but intermittent. In one case, they may also have indigestion, a tendency to loose stools, lack of warmth in their feet, red eyes, a dry mouth and desire for cold drinks, while the other person has a wet, weeping, crusty skin rash with red borders, a tendency to hay fever, ringing in their ears, and dizziness when they stand up. In Chinese medicine just as in modern Western medicine, both these patients suffer from headache. That is their disease diagnosis. However, they also suffer from a whole host of other complaints, have very different types of headaches, and very different constitutions, ages, and sex. In Chinese medicine, the patient's pattern is made up from all these other signs and symptoms and other information. Thus, in Chinese medicine, the pattern describes the totality of the person as a unique individual. And in Chinese medicine, treatment is designed to rebalance that entire pattern of imbalance as well as address the major complaint or disease. Thus, there is a saying in Chinese medicine:

One disease, different treatments
Different diseases, same treatment

This means that, in Chinese medicine, two patients with the same named disease diagnosis may receive different treatments if their Chinese medical patterns are different, while two patients diagnosed with different named diseases may receive the same treatment if their Chinese medical pattern is the same. In other words, in Chinese medicine, treatment is predicated primarily on one's pattern discrimination, not on one's named disease diagnosis. Therefore, each person is treated individually.

Since every patient gets just the treatment which is right to restore balance to their particular body, there are also no unwanted side effects. Side effects come from forcing one part of the body to behave while causing an imbalance in some other part. The medicine may have fit part of the problem but not the entirety of the patient as an individual. This is like robbing Peter to pay Paul. Since Chinese medicine sees the entire body (and mind!) as a single, unified whole, curing imbalance in one area of the body while causing it in another is unacceptable.

Below is a description of the major Chinese medical patterns at work in diabetes.

Treatment based on pattern discrimination

In the Chinese literature, the patterns of "flowing away and thirst" or "wasting and thirsting," depending on your translation, are usually arranged according to what are called the three burners. The three burners are three anatomical areas of the body. The upper burner refers to everything in the body above the diaphragm. However, in the case of diabetes, mainly refers to the lungs. The middle burner refers to everything in the body between the diaphragm and the navel. However, in terms of diabetes, mainly refers to the spleen and stomach. While the lower burner refers to everything below the navel, but, in the case of diabetes, mainly refers to the kidneys. Depending on which organs are involved, one then talks about upper wasting, middle wasting, lower wasting, and combinations of these.

Chinese and Western clinicians often refer to the three main symptoms of diabetes as the "three polys." These are polyphagia, meaning excessive eating, polydipsia, meaning excessive drinking, and polyuria, meaning excessive urination. In Chinese medicine, polyphagia is related to the stomach, polydipsia is related to the lungs, and polyuria is related to the kidneys. So polyphagia characterizes middle wasting, polydipsia characterizes upper wasting, and polyuria characterizes lower wasting.

Most modern Chinese clinicians agree that without some kind of evil heat, there is no diabetes. Then, depending on the patient's constitution, age, and other factors, such as diet and lifestyle, they may have a combination of upper and middle wasting, middle and lower wasting, or wasting of all three burners.

1. Upper wasting

This pattern is also referred to as lung heat with fluid damage.

Main symptoms: Vexatious thirst, copious drinking, a dry mouth, frequent, excessive urination, red tongue edges and tip with dry, thin, yellow coating, and a surging, rapid pulse

Treatment principles: Clear heat and moisten the lungs, engender fluids and relieve thirst

In actual fact, although the name of this pattern does not say so, the heat in the lungs has come from the stomach.

2. Middle wasting

This pattern is also referred to as stomach heat accumulation and exuberance.

Main symptoms: Excessive hunger, high food intake, emaciation, dry stools or constipation, thirst, a yellow tongue coating, and a slippery, forceful, probably rapid pulse

3. Lower wasting

Lower wasting is made up of two patterns, kidney yin debility and vacuity.and yin and yang dual vacuity.

A. Kidney yin debility & vacuity
Main symptoms: Frequent, profuse urination, turbid urination like grease or fat, possible sweet urination, a dry mouth and lips, a red tongue, and a deep, fine, rapid pulse

Treatment principles: Enrich yin and secure the kidneys

B. Yin & yang dual vacuity
Main symptoms: Frequent, numerous urination, turbid urination like fat, if severe, urinating every time one has a drink, a sooty, "black" facial complexion, dry, scorched rims of the ears or auricles, low back soreness, knee weakness, a cold body, fear of chill, possible impotence, a pale tongue with white coating, and a deep, fine, forceless pulse

Treatment principles: Warm yang, enrich the kidneys, and secure and contain (the urine)

While these are the main patterns described in the textbook literature under "flowing away and thirst" or "wasting and thirsting," real life is not so simple. In real-life patients, the above patterns are usually complicated by any of a large number of other patterns. Below are some of the most common of these.

1. Spleen qi vacuity

Main symptoms: Fatigue which is worse after large meals, lack of strength, a craving for sweets, possible obesity, abdominal distention after meals, a swollen tongue with teeth marks along its edges, possible cracks down its center or on its edges and a white coating, and a soggy pulse

Treatment principles: Fortify the spleen and boost the qi

Although the above signs and symptoms are the textbook signs and symptoms for this pure pattern, this pure pattern is never met in clinical practice. At the least, spleen qi vacuity is combined with stomach heat accumulation and exuberance.

2. Liver depression qi stagnation

Main symptoms: Irritability, premenstrual breast distention and pain, chest and side of the rib pain, lower abdominal distention and pain, discomfort in the stomach and epigastrium, diminished appetite, possible delayed menstruation whose amount is either scanty or profuse, darkish, stagnant menstrual blood, the menses unable to come easily, a normal or slightly dark tongue with thin, white coating, and a bowstring, fine pulse

Treatment principles: Course the liver and rectify the qi

This pattern likewise rarely occurs in the simple, textbook way presented above. However, it is also rare to find a patient with diabetes who does not have at least an element of liver depression. Because of the reciprocal relationship between the liver and spleen, when the liver gets depressed, the spleen tends to become vacuous and damp at the same time as the stomach tends to become hot and dry. Because the spleen engenders and transforms the blood, liver depression with spleen vacuity often gives rise to blood vacuity as well. If this pattern endures or due to aggravating circumstances, such as aging, menstruation, or lactation, it may also evolve into liver depression with yin vacuity failing to nourish the viscera, meaning primarily failing to nourish the heart viscus and the spirit the heart houses within it.

3. Liver depression transforming into heat

Main symptoms: All the signs and symptoms under the foregoing pattern plus the following: very easy anger, chest oppression, mental restlessness, insomnia, excessive dreams, red eyes, a red facial complexion, heart palpitations, a bitter taste in the mouth, and thirst. The tongue is red, perhaps with swollen edges, and a yellow coating. The pulse is bowstring and rapid.

Treatment principles: Course the liver and rectify the qi, clear heat and resolve depression

4. Liver qi invading the stomach

Main symptoms: All the signs and symptoms under pattern number two plus: epigastric and side of the rib distention and pain, nausea, vomiting, hiccup, and burping or belching. The tongue coating is thin and white, and the pulse is bowstring.

Treatment principles: Course the liver and rectify the qi, harmonize the stomach and downbear counterflow

5. Qi & yin dual vacuity

This is an abbreviation for spleen qi and kidney yin vacuity.

Main symptoms: The symptoms of this pattern depend on whether spleen qi or kidney yin is most vacuous. Symptoms of spleen qi vacuity include a sallow or pale complexion, reduced appetite, shortness of breath, weak limbs, fatigue, and disinclination to speak due to fatigue. Symptoms of kidney yin vacuity include flushed red cheeks in the afternoon or evening, tinnitus, dizziness, low back soreness, weak knees, and nocturia. The tongue in this case is swollen but red with a scanty, possibly white or yellow coating. If qi vacuity is more pronounced, the tongue may be simply pale with a red tip. The pulse tends to be fine, forceless, and rapid or large and vacuous.

Treatment principles: Supplement the qi and nourish yin

6. Heart-lung dual vacuity

This pattern describes a heart and lung qi and yin vacuity with vacuity heat.

Main symptoms: A pale complexion but flushed cheeks in the afternoon or early evening, lack of strength, spontaneous perspiration on slight exertion, and shortness of breath, anxiety, insomnia, heat in the palms and soles of the feet, a dry throat and tongue, heart palpitations, and impaired memory. The tongue is red, and the coating is thin and white. The pulse is fine and rapid.

Treatment principles: Supplement the and nourish yin, quiet the heart and secure the lungs

7. Heart-spleen dual vacuity

This pattern describes a heart blood and spleen qi vacuity.

Main symptoms: A pale complexion, forgetfulness, heart palpitations, dream-disturbed sleep, fatigue, lack of strength, poor appetite, a pale, swollen tongue with a thin, white coating, and a fine, forceless, slightly slow pulse. Because the spleen contains the blood within its vessels, this pattern is often complicated by various types of bleeding disorders. Therefore, women may have early periods with pale-colored, watery but profuse blood or continuous uterine bleeding with scanty flow.

Treatment principles: Supplement the heart and fortify the spleen, boost the qi and nourish the blood

8. Non-interaction of the heart & kidneys

Main symptoms: Vexation and agitation, vexatious heat in the center of the heart, restlessness, severe, continuous heart palpitations or racing heart, anxiety and forgetfulness, deafness, dizziness, sweating, coolness of the lower limbs, great difficulty falling asleep, a red tongue with a scanty coating or a bright red tongue, and a fine, rapid or surging pulse

Treatment principles: Clear the heart and lead yang to move downward to its lower origin

9. Liver blood vacuity

Main symptoms: Dizziness, blurred vision and especially night-blindness, anxiety and palpitations, insomnia, poor memory, headache, tingling and numbness of the extremities, stiffness of the joints with difficult bending and stretching, scanty menstruation, delayed menstruation, or amenorrhea, premature greying of the hair, pale or brittle nails, a pale red tongue with a thin, white coating, and a bowstring, fine pulse

Treatment principles: Supplement the liver and nourish the blood

10. Spleen-kidney yang vacuity

This pattern actually describes a spleen qi-kidney yang vacuity.

Main symptoms: Low back and knee soreness and weakness, chilled extremities and especially the feet, inhibited or excessive urination, nighttime urination, early morning diarrhea, loose stools, fatigue, lassitude of the spirit, generalized edema, dizziness standing up, infertility, a pale or dark, swollen tongue with teeth-marks and a white, slimy coating, and a deep, fine, forceless pulse

Treatment principles: Warm and supplement the spleen and kidneys

11. Blood stasis

Main symptoms: Premenstrual or menstrual lower abdominal pain which is either severe or is fixed in location and sharp or piercing in nature, varicose veins, chronic hemorrhoids, various types of lower abdominal lumps and masses, such as endometriosis, ovarian cysts, and uterine fibroids, lumps in the breast, sharp, piercing pain anywhere in the body which is fixed in location and which tends to be worse in the evenings and at night, a dark, dusky facial complexion or a tendency to brown spots on the skin, such as so-called age or liver spots, a purplish tongue or a tongue with static spots or static macules (*i.e.*, black and blue patches), dark, engorged, twisted and prominent veins under the tongue, and a bowstring, fine, choppy pulse

Treatment principles: Quicken the blood and transform or dispel stasis

This pattern is rarely encountered as the sole pattern accounting for a person's diabetes. Therefore, most clinical manuals do not even list it. However, blood stasis does commonly complicate many disorders, especially in women and in the elderly. In such cases, the treatment principles for blood stasis are then added to the other treatment principles, and the treatment for blood stasis is then added to other treatments for other patterns.

12. Phlegm dampness

Main symptoms: Excessive phlegm that is white in color and easily expectorated, chest and diaphragmatic oppression, nausea and vomiting, fatigue of the body and limbs, dizziness and vertigo, heart palpitations, a white, moist, slimy tongue coating, and a slippery pulse

Treatment principles: Dry dampness and transform phlegm, rectify the qi and harmonize the center

Harmonizing the center means to harmonize and regulate the upbearing and downbearing of the qi mechanism. The nausea and vomiting are all evidence that there is upward counterflow. Most commonly, this upward counterflow is due to liver depression qi stagnation resulting in counterflow. If qi backs up and accumulates, eventually it must vent itself somewhere. Since it is yang, it typically vents itself upward.

13. Phlegm heat

Main symptoms: Cough and rapid breathing with thick, yellow or white phlegm that is difficult to expectorate and may be flecked with blood, feverishness, dry throat, lips, and tongue, a red tongue with yellow coating, and a slippery, rapid pulse

Treatment principles: Dry dampness and transform phlegm, clear heat and harmonize the center

When there is enduring liver depressive or transformative heat or when yin vacuity heat is present, these may combine with phlegm dampness, producing phlegm heat. When phlegm heat is not cleared, it brews in the interior and can transform into fire.

The real deal

Although textbook discriminations such as the ones above make it seem like all the practitioner has to do is match up their patient's symptoms with one of the aforementioned patterns and then prescribe the recommended guiding formula, in actual clinical practice, one usually encounters combinations of the above discreet patterns and their related disease mechanisms. For instance, liver depression transforming heat may be complicated by spleen qi and heart blood vacuity. This, in turn may also be complicated by phlegm or blood stasis. Likewise, yin vacuity with fire effulgence may be complicated by liver depression and qi vacuity, liver depression and blood stasis, or liver depression and phlegm.

Although there are many patterns one may encounter in patients with either hypoglycemia or diabetes, the spleen and stomach sit squarely in the center of the disease mechanisms leading to diabetes. In this case, the stomach is typically hot and dry, thus damaging yin fluids, while the spleen is typically damp and weak. Mix in liver depression due to stress, kidney vacuity due to age, and blood stasis due to enduring disease and one has the most common disease mechanisms leading to this condition. Although there is little we can do about age itself, we do have control over what we eat and our lifestyles. Therefore, in order to prevent and treat diabetes, we should pay close attention to the main cause spleen-stomach imbalance—diet—and to the main cause of liver depression/depressive heat—stress.

How This System Works in Real-life

Using all the above information on the theory of Chinese medicine and the patterns and their mechanisms of diabetes, let's see how a Chinese doctor makes this system work in real-life.

Joanne's case

Take Joanne, for instance, whom I introduced at the beginning of this book. She has been having hypoglycemia for several months and could be considered pre-diabetic. Specifically, Joanne has been having trouble getting up in the morning. She has many disturbing dreams and is restless at night. Then, in the morning she is already fatigued even before the day begins. Joanne is 35 years old. She is somewhat overweight but has thought of herself as being in good health. When Joanne gets under stress, she often feels a lump in the back of her throat as if there was something there which she could neither swallow down nor spit up. She describes this as "postnasal drip" and says that she typically does hack up some white phlegm every morning when brushing her teeth. She also says that her limbs feel tight and tense, made worse by a stressful day at the office. Joanne also says that she often has headaches which make her face feel hot. Nothing over-the-counter helps these headaches; so she tries to sleep until they go away. Her chest feels stuffy and tight and she often sighs. When she really gets stressed, she feels some pain in her left chest or ribs. That scares her and she worries about having a heart attack. This fear of heart attack is worsened by the presence of heart palpitations when she gets nervous or doesn't eat meals. Joanne usually associates all these symptoms with the stress of her job, since everyone she knows at the office complains about the same sort of symptoms to a greater or lesser degree. Joanne thinks that this is the way that everyone is, that this is how you must inevitably feel when under stress.

Lately, Joanne has noticed that she is frequently getting red, painful gums and bad breath. When she does manage to get a full meal, she indulges in hot, spicy foods or foods that have rich sauces or gravy. She usually has a sticky or bitter taste in her mouth when she wakes up in the morning which is worse if she's eaten such a rich meal. Joanne's symptoms are always worse before her menstruation, at which time she also has sore, swollen breasts, lower abdominal distention, and a tendency to constipation which turns to diarrhea on the first day of her period. She has had moderately painful cramps on the first day of her period for years, but again, she has never discussed this with anyone because she thinks this is normal for women. Joanne has mood swings, is sometimes irritable and sometimes despondent, is fatigued, and feels weak in the limbs. Recently, she's noticed that her pale complexion and spontaneous perspiration have gotten worse especially after trying to satisfy her sugar cravings. When I ask her to stick out her tongue, it is somewhat redder than normal on its tip and edges. It has a pale center and a slightly yellow, somewhat slimy fur or coating. Her pulse is bowstring, slippery, and rapid.

How a Chinese doctor analyzes Joanne's symptoms

In Chinese medicine, fatigue, pale complexion, spontaneous perspiration, and weakness in the limbs is due to spleen qi vacuity. Joanne's slight obesity and excessive phlegm suggest that phlegm dampness is playing a part in her total pattern or picture. The feeling of phlegm in the back of her throat is called plum pit qi in Chinese medicine and is an indication of upwardly counterflowing phlegm lodged in the throat due to liver depression qi stagnation in turn due to stress. This is confirmed by Joanne's premenstrual breast distention and pain, tightness in the chest, premenstrual and menstrual lower abdominal pain, constipation before the onset of her menses, irritability, and bowstring pulse, all of which when taken together in Chinese medicine are seen as the hallmarks of liver depression qi stagnation. The bitter taste in her mouth in the morning shows that enduring liver depression has transformed into heat. This is confirmed by the red tongue tip and edges, the rapid pulse, the yellow tongue fur all indicating heat. The slimy fur and the slippery pulse indicate phlegm. The loose stools at the onset of the menses and the fatigue indicate that the phlegm is, in part, due to spleen qi vacuity not moving and transforming fluids which then gather and accumulate, first transforming into dampness and then congealing into phlegm. These spleen qi vacuity symptoms are especially pronounced after a period of eating poorly and eating too many refined sugars and carbohydrates. The fact that the palpitations occur at the same time indicates a spleen and heart vacuity relationship.

In the last chapter we discussed the disease mechanism of liver depression qi stagnation and its influence on the spleen and stomach. In Joanne's case, both the spleen and stomach are affected. The frontal headaches, the sore, painful gums, the bad breath, and the restless night after evening meals which are hot and spicy, all indicate an element of stomach heat. This stomach heat is made worse by the horizontal movement of the liver's depressive heat. Therefore, the Chinese doctor knows that there is a combination of liver depression transforming heat and spleen vacuity engendering dampness and then phlegm. This is complicated by stomach heat and a disharmony between the spleen and the heart. Joanne's Western doctor tells her that she has an early case on non-insulin dependent diabetes (NIDD).[4]

---

[4] Chinese medicine can often cure NIDD. Although it is generally agreed that Chinese medicine cannot cure IDD or insulin-dependent diabetes, Chinese medicine can help slow down and eliminate the symptoms of deterioration associated with this form of diabetes.

How a Chinese doctor treats Joanne's diabetes

Once a Chinese doctor knows the patient's pattern discrimination, the next step is to formulate the treatment principles necessary to rebalance the imbalance implied by this pattern dis-crimination. If the Chinese doctor listed liver depression, spleen vacuity as the main pattern, then the treatment principles are to course the liver and rectify qi, fortify the spleen and boost the qi. If the Chinese doctor said that, secondarily, there is liver depressive heat attacking the stomach, then they would add the principles of clearing liver-stomach heat and harmonizing the stomach. Further, if phlegm is due to spleen vacuity not moving and transforming body fluids, then one should also dry dampness and transform phlegm. Lastly, since spleen vacuity is affecting the heart, then the Chinese doctor would supplement the heart and nourish the blood.

Once the Chinese doctor has stated these treatment principles, then they know that anything which works to accomplish these principles will be good for the patient. Using these principles, the Chinese doctor can now select various acupuncture points which achieve these effects. They can prescribe Chinese herbal medicinals which embody these principles. They can make recommendations about what to eat and not eat based on these principles. They can make recommendations on lifestyle changes. And, in short, they can advise the patient on any and every aspect of their life, judging whether something either aids the accomplishment of these principles or works against it.

In Chinese medicine, the internal administration of Chinese "herbal" medicinals is the main modality.[5] So let's look at how a

---

[5] I say herbal in quotation marks because the word herbal implies medicinals from vegetable sources. But Chinese medicinals come from all three realms: vegetable, mineral, and animal. Therefore, the word herbal is actually a misnomer.

Chinese doctor crafts a prescription for Joanne. Because the first treatment principle stated for Joanne is to course the liver and rectify the qi, fortify the spleen and harmonize the constructive, the Chinese doctor knows that he or she should select their guiding formula from the harmonizing and resolving category of formulas. Depending on the textbook, there are 22-28 main categories of formulas in Chinese medicine, each category correlated to a main treatment principle. The category of harmonizing and resolving formulas is subdivided into formulas which harmonize the liver and spleen, the liver and stomach, the stomach and intestines, or the *shao yang*.[6] Since Joanne's case has to do first with liver depression, spleen vacuity, we need to pick a formula from those which course the liver and fortify the spleen.

Under this category of formulas, there are some formulas which mainly treat hepatitis, gastritis, menopausal syndromes, anemia, and other gynecological complaints. Since Joanne's main complaint is fatigue and weakness, we must look for a formula which is empirically known through clinical experience to treat fatigue due to spleen vacuity. Very quickly the list narrows down to one very famous formula, *Xiao Yao San* (Rambling Powder). This formula is for the treatment of fatigue, headache, distended breasts and other symptoms of premenstrual syndrome due to liver depression and spleen vacuity with an element of blood vacuity. Since liver depression is already a part of this formula's rationale, we may not need to add anything more for the liver depression qi stagnation that we have identified earlier. However, this formula does not include anything for clearing depressive heat or harmonizing the stomach. Therefore, we will have to add some ingredients for these purposes.

---

[6] The *shao yang* refers to a condition where an externally invading pathogen is half on the inside of the body and half still in the exterior or relative outside of the body. It describes a stage in certain types of externally contracted diseases, such as colds and flues.

Hence the final formula composed by the Chinese doctor will be called *Xiao Yao San Jia Jian* (Rambling Powder with Additions & Subtractions). This formula might be comprised of:

Radix Bupleuri (*Chai Hu*)
Radix Angelicae Sinensis (*Dang Gui*)
Radix Paeoniae Lactiflorae (*Bai Shao*)
Rhizoma Atractylodes Macrocephalae (*Bai Zhu*)
Sclerotium Poriae Cocos (*Fu Ling*)
honey-fried Radix Glycyrrhizae (*Gan Cao*)
Radix Codonopsitis Pilosulae (*Dang Shen*)
Radix Astragali Membranacei (*Huang Qi*)
Tuber Ophiopogonis Japonici (*Mai Dong*)
Rhizoma Anemarrhenae Aspheloidis (*Zhi Mu*)
Radix Trichosanthis Kirlowii (*Tian Hua Fen*)
Radix Scutellariae Baicalensis (*Huang Qin*)
Rhizoma Pinelliae Ternatae (*Ban Xia*)
Pericarpium Citri Reticulatae (*Chen Pi*)
Fructus Zizyphi Jujubae (*Da Zao*)

Bupleurum courses the liver and resolves depression. Dang Gui and Peony nourish the blood and soften (*i.e.,* relax) the liver. Atractylodes and Poria fortify the spleen and eliminate dampness. On the one hand, they promote the movement and transformation of liqiuds, while, on the other, promote the engenderment and transformation of the qi. Codonopsis and Astragalus fortify the spleen and boost the qi, specifically treating the fatigue and lethargy. Honey-fried Licorice boosts the qi and supplements the center while nourishing the heart and quieting the spirit. Scutellaria is the main ingredient for clearing depressive heat from the stomach and liver. It is assisted in clearing by Trichosanthes, Ophiopogon, and Anemarrhena. These latter three medicinals all clear heat in the stomach and engender fluids, thus treating a dry mouth and thirst. They are very common ingredients in formulas for diabetics since thirst is such a common symptom of diabetes. In addition, both Trichosanthes and Ophiopogon transform phlegm. Pinellia and Citrus Peel (*i.e.,*

Chen Pi), dry dampness, transform phlegm, harmonize the stomach and downbear counterflow. And Red Dates (*Zizyphus*) fortify the spleen, nourish the heart, and harmonize all the other medicinals in the formula, helping to insure that none of them cause any unwanted side effects.[7]

Hence one can see that the ingredients in this formula very precisely and specifically embody and carry out the treatment principles we have said were necessary for rebalancing Joanne's condition. To make this formula even more effective, the Chinese doctor will modify it further from week to week as Joanne's symptoms change and as she moves through her menstrual cycle. For instance, since Joanne experiences premenstrual symptoms with breast distention and tightness in the chest, during her premenstruum, I might add Rhizoma Cyperi Rotundi (*Xiang Fu*) and Tuber Curcumae (*Yu Jin*) to further move the qi and disperse distention. These would also help the menstrual cramps.

Usually, a formula such as this would be taken two to three times each day. The herbs would be soaked in water and then boiled into a very strong "tea" for 30-45 minutes. Each week, I would check with Joanne to see how she was doing and if I needed to make any modifications to her formula. Remember, the Chinese doctor wants to heal without causing any side effects. If the formula does cause any unwanted effects, then it is my job to add and subtract ingredients until it achieves a perfect result with no unwanted effects.

The ingredients in this formula may also be taken as a dried, powdered extract. Such extracts are manufactured by several Taiwanese and Japanese companies. Although such extracts are not, in my experience, as powerful as the freshly decocted "teas",

---

[7] As this formula is written here, it is actually a combination of three famous formulas: *Xiao Yao San* (Rambling Powder), *Xiao Chai Hu Tang* (Minor Bupleurum Decoction), and *Er Chen Tang* (Two Aged [Ingredients] Decoction) with other modifications.

they are easier to take. Many standard formulas also come as ready-made pills. However, these cannot be modified. If their ingredients match the individual patient's requirements, then they are fine. If the formula needs modifications, then teas or powders whose individual ingredients can be added and subtracted are necessary.

In exactly the same way, the Chinese doctor could create an individualized acupuncture treatment plan and would certainly create an accompanying dietary and lifestyle plan. However, we will discuss each of these in their own chapter. In a woman Joanne's age with her Chinese pattern discrimination, either Chinese herbal medicine alone, acupuncture alone, or a combination of the two supported by the proper diet and lifestyle will usually eliminate or at the very least drastically diminish her symptoms within two to three weeks. Often results will be apparent within the first few days after beginning the herbs, for instance in symptoms such as thirst and fatigue.

And when Chinese medicine gets its results, it does so without side effects. If the patient tells their practitioner that they are having some side effects from their Chinese medicinals, then the Chinese medical practitioner must adjust the formula, adding and subtracting ingredients, until the healing effects are obtained while the side effects are eliminated. Since the entire body is seen in Chinese medicine as a unified, integrated whole, trying to cure while causing side effects is like robbing Peter to pay Paul. It cannot result in true health.

Chinese Herbal Medicine & Diabetes

As we have seen from Joanne's case above, there is no Chinese "diabetes herb" or even a "diabetes formula" which will work for all sufferers of this disease. Chinese medicinals are individually prescribed based on a person's pattern discrimination, not on a disease diagnosis like diabetes. Patients often come to me and say, "My friend told me that *Si Jun Zi Wan* (Four Gentleman Pills, a common Chinese over-the-counter medication) is good for fatigue and lack of strength. But I tried it and it didn't work." This is because *Si Jun Zi Wan* is meant to treat a specific pattern of fatigue, not fatigue *per se*. If you exhibit that pattern, then this formula will work. If you do not have the signs and symptoms of this pattern, it won't.

In addition, because most people's diabetic condition is a combination of different Chinese patterns and disease mechanisms, professional Chinese medicine never treats diabetes with herbal "singles." In herbalism, singles mean the prescription of a single herb all by itself. Chinese herbal medicine is based on rebalancing patterns, and patterns in real-life patients almost always have more than a single element. Therefore, Chinese doctors almost always prescribe herbs in multi-ingredient formulas. Such formulas may have anywhere from 6 to 18 or more ingredients. When a Chinese doctor reads a prescription by another Chinese doctor, they can tell you not only what the patient's pattern discrimination is, but also their probable signs and symptoms. In other words, the Chinese doctor does not just combine several medicinals which are all reputed to be "good for

diabetes." Rather, they carefully craft a formula whose ingredients are meant to rebalance every aspect of the patient's
body-mind.

Getting your own individualized prescription

Since, in China, it takes not less than four years of full-time
college education to learn how to do a professional Chinese
pattern discrimination and then write an herbal formula based on
that pattern discrimination, most laypeople cannot realistically
write their own Chinese herbal prescriptions. It should also be
remembered that Chinese herbs are not effective and safe
because they are either Chinese or herbal. In fact, approximately
20% of the common Chinese materia medica did not originate in
Chinese, and not all Chinese herbs are completely safe. They are
only safe when prescribed according to a correct pattern discrimination, in the right dose, and for the right amount of time.
After all, if an herb is strong enough to heal an imbalance, it is
also strong enough to create an imbalance if overdosed or
misprescribed. Therefore, I strongly recommend persons who
wish to experience the many benefits of Chinese herbal medicine
to see a qualified professional practitioner who can do a
professional pattern discrimination and write you an individualized prescription. Towards the end of this book, I will give the
reader suggestions on how to find a qualified professional Chinese
medical practitioner near you.

Experimenting with Chinese patent medicines

In reality, qualified professional practitioners of Chinese medicine are not yet found in every Western community. In addition,
some people may want to try to heal their diabetes as much on
their own as possible. More and more health food stores are
stocking a variety of ready-made Chinese formulas in pill and
powder form. These ready-made, over-the-counter Chinese
medicines are often referred to as Chinese patent medicines.
Although my best recommendation is for readers to seek Chinese
herbal treatment from professional practitioners, below are some

suggestions of how one might experiment with Chinese patent medicines to treat diabetes.

In chapter 5, I have given the signs and symptoms of the five key patterns associated with most people's diabetes. These are:

1. Lung heat damaging fluids
2. Stomach heat accumulation & exuberance
3. Kidney yin vacuity
4. Yin & yang vacuity

Then I have gone on to discuss several other patterns which, while they are usually not discussed in Chinese textbooks on diabetes *per se*, commonly complicate most diabetic patients' patterns. These are:

1. Spleen qi vacuity
2. Liver depression
3. Depressive heat
4. Qi & yin dual vacuity
5. Blood stasis
6. Phlegm dampness or phlegm heat

If the reader can identify their main and complicating patterns from chapter 5, then there are some Chinese patent remedies that they might consider trying. Even if one can only identify their main pattern and take the formula for that main pattern, they should experience some benefit. The names and addresses of suppliers of these Chinese patent medicines are given in the back of this book.

Qing Zao Jiu Fei Tang Lung Heat

Qing Zao Jiu Fei Tang means Clear Dryness & Rescue the Lungs Decoction. Although its name contains the word decoction, this formula is now available in pill form. This formula is very effective for clearing heat from the lungs and engendering fluids in both the lungs and stomach. Therefore, although this formula is mostly thought of as a remedy for chronic bronchitis and asthma, it can be used for the pattern of lung heat damaging fluids.

The ingredients in this formula are:

Gypsum Fibrosum (*Shi Gao*)
Tuber Ophiopogonis Japonici (*Mai Men Dong*)
Folium Eriobotryae Japonicae (*Pi Pa Ye*)
Radix Panacis Ginseng (*Ren Shen*)
Gelatinum Corii Asini (*E Jiao*)
Folium Mori Albi (*Sang Ye*)
Semen Pruni Armeniacae (*Xing Ren*)
Radix Glycyrrhizae (*Gan Cao*)
Semen Lini Usitatissimi (*Hu Ma Ren*)

Gypsum clears heat and drains fire from the stomach and lungs. Ophiopogon enriches yin and engenders fluids in the stomach and lungs. It also clears heat and transforms phlegm. Eriobotrya clears heat from the stomach and lungs, transforms phlegm, and downbears counterflow of the stomach and lungs. Ginseng supplements the qi and engenders fluids. It strongly fortifies the spleen qi, but also supplements the qi of all five viscera. Folium Mori dispels wind and clears heat from the lungs. However, it does this without being drying, since it is indicated for lung dryness conditions. Armeniaca mainly stops cough and transforms phlegm. However, it also moistens the intestines and engenders fluids. Licorice helps Ginseng supplement the spleen and boost the qi. It also clears heat and engenders some fluids. And Semen Linum or Linseed moistens the intestines and engenders fluids as well.

Sha Shen Mai Dong Tang Dryness (Qi is OK)

This medicine's name translates as Glehnia & Ophiopogon Decoction, and, once again, although its name contains the word decoction, it is available in pill form. This formula also treats lung and stomach fluid dryness where there is not as much heat. Since heat does complicate most diabetics' scenarios, this formula would typically be combined with some other formula or formulas. Like the above formula, it does supplement the spleen at least a bit. Its ingredients are:

Semen Dolichoris Lablab (*Bai Bian Dou*)
Radix Trichosanthis Kirlowii (*Tian Hua Fen*)
Folium Mori Albi (*Sang Ye*)
Rhizoma Polygonati Odorati (*Yu Zhu*)
Tuber Ophiopogon Japonici (*Mai Dong*)
Radix Glehniae Littoralis (*Sha Shen*)
Radix Glycyrrhizae (*Gan Cao*)

This formula contains some of the same ingredients as the one above. Of those that are different, Dolichos clears damp heat without being drying at the same time as it fortifies the spleen. Trichosanthes clears heat from the stomach and lungs while engendering fluids. It is a very important Chinese medicinal for treating dry mouth and thirst. Polygonatum Odoratum nourishes yin and moistens dryness in the lungs and stomach. It also extinguishes wind and moistens the sinews. Internal wind and malnourishment of the sinews are often to blame for diabetic symptoms such as itching of the skin and numbness and tingling of the extremities. Glehnia supplements the lungs and enriches yin, supplementing the qi as well as engendering fluids.

Bai He Gu Jin Wan Lu, St, Ki Yin def signs

Bai He Gu Jin Wan or Lily Bulb Secure Metal Pills is also a formula which is mostly used for chronic bronchitis and asthma. However, because it contains a number of medicinals that nourish and enrich stomach, lung, and kidney yin, it can be used to treat lung yin fluid dryness patterns of this disease. Its heat-clearing and spleen-supplementing abilities are weak. So you will probably want to combine it with some other formula or formulas. Its ingredients are:
Bulbus Lilii (*Bai He*)

uncooked Radix Rehmanniae (*Sheng Di*)
Radix Rehmanniae (*Shu Di*)
Tuber Ophiopogonis Japonici (*Mai Men Dong*)
Radix Scrophulariae Ninpoensis (*Xuan Shen*)
Bulbus Fritillariae (*Bei Mu*)
Radix Platycodi Grandiflori (*Jie Geng*)
Radix Angelicae Sinensis (*Dang Gui*)
Radix Albus Paeoniae Lactiflorae (*Bai Shao*)
Radix Glycyrrhizae (*Gan Cao*)

Yu Quan Wan

Yu Quan Wan means Jade Spring Pills. It is a famous Chinese patent medicine which has been designed specifically to treat "flowing away and thirst" or "wasting and thirsting disease" due to lung, stomach, and kidney yin vacuity complicated by spleen qi vacuity and lung-stomach heat. Its ingredients include:

Radix Trichosanthis Kirlowii (*Tian Hua Fen*)
Fructus Germinatus Hordei Vulgaris (*Mai Ya*)
Sclerotium Poriae Cocos (*Fu Ling*)
Radix Astragali Membranacei (*Huang Qi*)
Radix Glycyrrhizae (*Gan Cao*)
uncooked Radix Rehmanniae (*Sheng Di*)
Radix Puerariae (*Ge Gen*)
Radix Codonopsitis Pilosulae (*Dang Shen*)
Fructus Pruni Mume (*Wu Mei*)
Fructus Schisandrae Chinensis (*Wu Wei Zi*)

Although this formula does not clear heat very effectively, it does a good job with the spleen qi and yin vacuity part of diabetes. It can be combined with other Chinese herbal remedies when clearing heat or addressing other disease mechanisms become necessary. For instance, it could be combined with the following formula.

Bai Hu Tang Jia Ren Shen

Bai hu means white tiger. So the name of this ready-made medicine is White Tiger Decoction and it too comes as a pill. It is indicated for stomach heat accumulation and exuberance. Its ingredients include:

Gypsum Fibrosum (*Shi Gao*)
Rhizoma Anemarrhenae Aspheloidis (*Zhi Mu*)] LARGOE IF W/constipation
Radix Dioscoreae Oppositae (*Shan Yao*)
mix-fried Radix Glycyrrhizae (*Gan Cao*)

HUANG QI

Within this modification of a very famous standard Chinese formula, Gyspum and Anemarrhena are combined to clear heat and engender fluids. This is a well-known pair for treating thirst due to heat in the stomach damaging yin fluids. Dioscorea supplements both the spleen and kidneys without being either overly drying or overly warming. It is a quite clever modification of this formula. Mix-fried Licorice also supplements the spleen while still engendering some fluids. It also nourishes the heart and quiets the spirit.

Liu Wei Di Huang Wan

This formula, whose name means Six Flavors Rehmannia Pills, nourishes liver blood and kidney yin. It is the primary formula to treat symptoms of yin vacuity. Its ingredients are:

cooked Radix Rehmanniae (*Shu Di*)
Fructus Corni Officinalis (*Shan Zhu Yu*)
Radix Dioscoreae Oppositae (*Shan Yao*)
Rhizoma Alismatis (*Ze Xie*)
Sclerotium Poriae Cocos (*Fu Ling*)
Cortex Radicis Moutan (*Dan Pi*)

In a very few people, one of the ingredients, Rehmannia, can cause diarrhea. If these pills cause diarrhea, their use should be stopped immediately.

This formula is a common one prescribed to diabetics in China if they suffer from the pattern of kidney yin vacuity. It can either be used alone or combined with other Chinese patent pills. Since most cases of diabetes include a substantial element of heat and this formula does not really clear any heat, the following modification of this formula is also commonly prescribed to diabetics.

Zhi Bai Di Huang Wan

Called Anemarrhena & Phellodendron Rehmannia Pills in English, these pills are made by adding two ingredients to the preceding formula. These two ingredients are:

Rhizoma Anemarrhenae Aspheloidis (*Zhi Mu*)
Cortex Phellodendri (*Huang Bai*)

Anemarrhena enriches kidney yin and clears vacuity heat, while Phellodendron clears vacuity heat from the upper body and damp heat from the lower body. Anemarrhena is a major Chinese herb for treating thirst, one of the main symptoms of diabetes. Signs of increased heat include night sweats, flushed red cheeks in the afternoon or evening, a red tongue with scanty, yellow coating, red rashes on the skin, and a rapid pulse.

Qi Ju Di Huang Wan

This formula is also derived from *Liu Wei Di Huang Wan* above by adding two other ingredients:

Fructus Lycii Chinensis (*Gou Qi Zi*)
Flos Chrysanthemi Morifolii (*Ju Hua*)

This then is called *Qi Ju Di Huang Wan* or Lycium & Chrysanthemum Rehmannia Pills. This formula is used for vision problems due to kidney yin and liver blood vacuity. Symptoms may include blurry vision, dry and painful eyes, pressure behind the eyes, and poor night vision. In this case, this formula may be useful in diabetic retinopathy. It is also used for sinews which lack malnourishment, and two of the symptoms which indicate such lack of nourishment of the sinews are numbness and tingling of the extremities, as in diabetic peripheral neuropathy or polyneuritis.

You Gui Wan

The name of these pills translates as Restore the Right Pills. This is because kidney yang is often referred to as the right kidney. This formula, therefore, is for the treatment of kidney yang vacuity. If there are no cold symptoms, such as cold feet, chilly, weak low back, copious, clear, nighttime urination, or decreased sexual desire, one should *not* use this formula. One should also suspend its use if it produces any symptoms of pathological heat. These might include sores on the tongue or in the mouth, sore throat, fever, or flu-like symptoms. This formula's ingredients include:

cooked Radix Rehmanniae (*Shu Di*)
Radix Lateralis Praeparatus Aconiti Carmichaeli (*Fu Zi*)
Cortex Cinnamomi Cassiae (*Rou Gui*)
Fructus Corni Officinalis (*Shan Zhu Yu*)
Fructus Lycii Chinensis (*Gou Qi Zi*)
Radix Dioscoreae Oppositae (*Shan Yao*)
Cortex Eucommiae Ulmoidis (*Du Zhong*)
Radix Angelicae Sinensis (*Dang Gui*)
Semen Cuscutae Chinensis (*Tu Si Zi*)
Gelatinum Cornu Cervi (*Lu Jiao Jiao*)

In actuality, this formula treats both kidney yin and yang vacuities, so it might be used for that pattern. However, it does not clear any heat. In that case, as is the case with most diabetics, one might consider combining this formula with *Zhi Bai Di Huang Wan* described above.

Jin Gui Shen Qi Wan

Jin Gui is an allusion to the name of the book this formula is taken from, *The Golden Cabinet*, a book written approximately 250 CE. The rest of the name means "kidney qi pills." Along with the preceding formula, this is one of the most famous formulas for supplementing kidney yang in Chinese medicine. In actuality, it supplements both kidney yin and yang since it is merely a modification of *Liu Wei Di Huang Wan* discussed above. The same caveats and cautions apply to its use. Its ingredients consist of:

cooked Radix Rehmanniae (*Shu Di*)
Radix Lateralis Praeparatus Aconiti Carmichaeli (*Fu Zi*)
Cortex Cinnamomi Cassiae (*Rou Gui*)
Fructus Corni Officinalis (*Shan Zhu Yu*)
Radix Dioscoreae Oppositae (*Shan Yao*)
Sclerotium Poriae Cocos (*Fu Ling*)
Rhizoma Alismatis (*Ze Xie*)
Cortex Radicis Moutan (*Dan Pi*)

Bu Zhong Yi Qi Wan

The name of this formula translates as Supplement the Center & Boost the Qi Pills. It strongly supplements spleen vacuity. It is commonly used to treat central qi fall, *i.e.*, prolapse of the stomach, uterus, or rectum due to spleen qi vacuity. However, it is a very complex formula with a very wide range of indications. It supplements the spleen but also courses the liver and rectifies the qi. It is one of the most commonly prescribed of all Chinese herbal formulas and these pills can be combined with a number of others when spleen qi vacuity plays a significant role in someone's condition. Its ingredients are:

Radix Astragali Membranacei (*Huang Qi*)
Radix Panacis Ginseng (*Ren Shen*)
Radix Glycyrrhizae (*Gan Cao*)
Rhizoma Atractylodis Macrocephalae (*Bai Zhu*)
Radix Angelicae Sinensis (*Dang Gui*)
Pericarpium Citri Reticulatae (*Chen Pi*)

Rhizoma Cimicifugae (*Sheng Ma*)
Radix Bupleuri (*Chai Hu*)
Rhizoma Atractylodis Macrocephalae (*Bai Zhu*)

This formula also does not include any heat-clearing medicinals and it tends to be drying. Therefore, most diabetics would want to combine this formula with one or more other pills which do clear heat or engender fluids. For instance, this formula might be combined with either *Zhi Bai Di Huang Wan* or *Qing Zao Jiu Fei Tang* (tablets).

Xiao Yao Wan

Xiao Yao Wan is one of the most common Chinese herbal formulas prescribed. Its Chinese name has been translated as Free & Easy Pills, Rambling Pills, Relaxed Wanderer Pills, and several other versions of this same idea of promoting a freer and smoother, more relaxed flow. As a patent medicine, this formula comes as pills, and there are both Chinese-made and American-made versions of this formula available over-the-counter in the Western marketplace. The ingredients in this formula are:

Radix Bupleuri (*Chai Hu*)
Radix Angelicae Sinensis (*Dang Gui*)
Radix Albus Paeoniae Lactiflorae (*Bai Shao*)
Rhizoma Atractylodis Macrocephalae (*Bai Zhu*)
Sclerotium Poriae Cocos (*Fu Ling*)
mix-fried Radx Glycyrrhizae (*Gan Cao*)
Herba Menthae Haplocalycis (*Bo He*)
uncooked Rhizoma Zingiberis (*Sheng Jiang*)

This formula treats the pattern of liver depression qi stagnation complicated by blood vacuity and spleen weakness with possible dampness as well. Bupleurum courses the liver and rectifies the qi. It is aided in this by Herba Menthae Haplocalycis or Peppermint. Dang Gui and Peony nourish the blood and soften and harmonize the liver. Atractylodes and Poria fortify the spleen and eliminate dampness. Mix-fried Licorice aids these two in fortifying the spleen and supplementing the liver, while uncooked Ginger aids in both promoting and regulating the qi flow and eliminating dampness.

This formula is also not usually thought of as a diabetic remedy and will need to be combined with some other Chinese patent pill in most cases of diabetes. However, when diabetes presents with the signs and symptoms of liver depression, spleen qi vacuity, and an element of blood vacuity, one can try taking this formula along with one or more others. If one notices any side effects after taking these pills at the dose recommended on the package, then stop immediately and seek a professional consultation. Such side effects from this formula might include nervousness, irritability, a dry mouth and increased thirst, and red, dry eyes. Such side effects show that this formula, at least without modification, is not right for you. Although it may be doing you some good, it is also causing some harm. Remember, Chinese medicine is meant to cure without side effects, and as long as the prescription matches one's pattern there will not be any.

Dan Zhi Xiao Yao Wan

Dan Zhi Xiao Yao Wan or Moutan & Gardenia Rambling Pills is a modification of the above formula which also comes as a patent medicine in the form of pills. It is meant to treat the pattern of liver depression transforming into heat with spleen vacuity and possible blood vacuity and/or dampness. The ingredients in this formula are the same as above except that two other herbs are added:

Cortex Radicis Moutan (*Dan Pi*)
Fructus Gardeniae Jasminoidis (*Shan Zhi Zi*)

These two ingredients clear heat and resolve depression. In addition, Cortex Radicis Moutan or Moutan quickens the blood and dispels stasis and is good at clearing heat specifically from the blood.

84

Basically, the signs and symptoms of the pattern for which this formula is designed are the same as those for *Xiao Yao San* above plus signs and symptoms of depressive heat. These might include a reddish tongue with a slightly yellow coating, a bowstring and rapid pulse, a bitter taste in the mouth, and increased irritability. Just as diabetics generally would not take *Xiao Yao Wan* alone, so this formula should most probably be combined with another Chinese patent pill. In that case, one might choose either to clear more heat or to nourish and enrich yin fluids.

Xiao Chai Hu Tang Wan

Meaning Minor Bupleurum Decoction Pills, this is the single most commonly prescribed Chinese herbal formula in the world. It is indicated for the treatment of liver depression with depressive heat in the liver, gallbladder, stomach, and/or lungs, spleen qi vacuity, and either stomach disharmony or phlegm. Its ingredients include:

Radix Bupleuri (*Chai Hu*)
Radix Codonopsitis Pilosulae (*Dang Shen*)
Radix Scutellariae Baicalensis (*Huang Qin*)
Rhizoma Pinelliae Ternatae (*Ban Xia*)
mix-fried Radix Glycyrrhizae (*Gan Cao*)
Fructus Zizyphi Jujubae (*Da Zao*)
uncooked Rhizoma Zingiberis (*Sheng Jiang*)

Like *Xiao Yao Wan* above, this formula is not usually discussed in Chinese herbal textbooks for wasting and thirsting, and for this condition would not be prescribed alone. However, since most diabetics do have elements of spleen vacuity and liver depression and since most diabetics do have heat in their stomachs, this formula can be used for diabetics when it is combined with other Chinese patent medicines which either clear heat more or enrich and engender yin fluids more.

Within this formula, Bupleurum courses the liver and rectifies the qi. Codonopsis, Licorice, and Red Dates all fortify the spleen and supplement the qi. Red Dates and Licorice also nourish the blood and calm the spirit. Scutellaria clears heat from the liver, gallbladder, stomach, and lungs. And uncooked Ginger transforms dampness, harmonizes the stomach, and assists in the movement of qi.

Tian Wang Bu Xin Dan

The name of this formula translates as Heavenly Emperor Supplement the Heart Elixir. It treats insomnia, restlessness, fatigue, and heart palpitations due to yin, blood, and qi vacuity, with an emphasis on heart yin and liver blood vacuity. Its ingredients include:

uncooked Radix Rehmanniae (*Sheng Di*)
Radix Scrophulariae Ningpoensis (*Xuan Shen*)
Fructus Schisandrae Chinensis (*Wu Wei Zi*)
Tuber Asparagi Cochinensis (*Tian Men Dong*)
Tuber Ophiopogonis Japonici (*Mai Men Dong*)
Radix Angelicae Sinensis (*Dang Gui*)
Semen Biotae Orientalis (*Bai Zi Ren*)
Semen Zizyphi Spinosae (*Suan Zao Ren*)
Radix Salviae Miltiorrhizae (*Dan Shen*)
Radix Polygalae Tenuifoliae (*Yuan Zhi*)
Sclerotium Poriae Cocos (*Fu Ling*)
Radix Codonopositis Pilosulae (*Dang Shen*)

There are five ingredients in this formula which are very effective for treating yin vacuity dryness leading to thirst. These are Rehmannia, Scrophularia, Schisandra, Asparagus, and Ophiopogon. This formula is not very strong at clearing heat. It does supplement the spleen qi, it does quicken the blood, and it does rectify the qi.

Ba Zhen Wan

Si Jun Zi T (Qi)
Si Wu T (BID)

Ba Zhen Wan or Eight Pearls Pills are prescribed for qi and blood dual vacuity. This formula boosts the qi and nourishes the blood whenever there is a spleen qi vacuity which has led to the qi being too weak and the blood insufficient. It can be used for fatigue, dizziness, heart palpitations, poor appetite, shortness of breath, a pale complexion, pale nails, a swollen, pale tongue with teeth-marks on its edges and a white coating, and a fine, weak pulse. Its ingredients are:

Radix Codonopositis Pilosulae (*Dang Shen*)
Radix Atractylodis Macrocephalae (*Bai Zhu*)
Sclerotium Poriae Cocos (*Fu Ling*)
mix-fried Radix Glycyrrhizae (*Gan Cao*)
cooked Radix Rehmanniae (*Shu Di*)
Radix Angelicae Sinensis (*Dang Gui*)
Radix Albus Paeoniae Lactiflorae (*Bai Shao*)
Radix Ligustici Wallichii (*Chuan Xiong*)

Gui Pi Wan

Gui means to return or restore, *pi* means the spleen, and *wan* means pills. Therefore, the name of these pills means Restore the Spleen Pills. However, these pills not only supplement the spleen qi but also nourish heart blood and calm the heart spirit. They are the textbook guiding formula for the pattern of heart-spleen dual vacuity. In this case, there are symptoms of spleen qi vacuity, such as fatigue, poor appetite, and cold hands and feet plus symptoms of heart blood vacuity, such as a pale tongue, heart palpitations, and insomnia. This formula is also the standard one for treating heavy or abnormal bleeding due to the spleen not containing and restraining the blood within its vessels. It does not clear any heat. It can be combined with *Xiao Chai Hu Tang* when there is liver depression/depressive heat complicated by heart blood and spleen qi vacuity. Its ingredients are:

Radix Astragali Membranacei (*Huang Qi*)
Radix Codonopsitis Pilosulae (*Dang Shen*)
Rhizoma Atractylodis Macrocephalae (*Bai Zhu*)
Sclerotium Parardicis Poriae Cocos (*Fu Shen*)
mix-fried Radix Glycyrrhizae (*Gan Cao*)
Radix Angelicae Sinensis (*Dang Gui*)

Semen Zizyphi Spinosae (*Suan Zao Ren*)
Arillus Euphoriae Longanae (*Long Yan Rou*)
Gelatinum Corii Asini (*E Jiao*)
Radix Polygalae Tenuifoliae (*Yuan Zhi*)
Radix Auklandiae Lappae (*Mu Xiang*)

Xue Fu Zhu Yu Wan

The name of these pills in English is Blood Mansion Dispel Stasis Pills. They are a commonly used basic formula for the treatment of blood stasis conditions. They can either be used as the main treatment for a predominately blood stasis pattern, or they can be combined with other Chinese patent medicines when blood stasis plays a contributory role. Remember, blood stasis pain is fixed in one spot, is typically severe, and often described as sharp, piercing, or stabbing. One should also remember the saying, "Enduring disease enters the network vessels." This means that chronic diseases are often complicated by blood stasis. Many Chinese clinicians assume that there is blood stasis complicating all cases of diabetic peripheral neuropathy. The ingredients in this formula consist of:

Semen Pruni Persicae (*Tao Ren*)
Flos Carthami Tinctorii (*Hong Hua*)
Radix Angelicae Sinensis (*Dang Gui*)
Radix Ligustici Wallichii (*Chuan Xiong*)
Radix Rubrus Paeoniae Lactiflorae (*Chi Shao*)
Radix Bupleuri (*Chai Hu*)
Radix Platycodi Grandiflori (*Jie Geng*)
Fructus Citri Aurantii (*Zhi Ke*)
uncooked Radix Rehmanniae (*Sheng Di*)
Radix Glycyrrhizae (*Gan Cao*)

Interestingly, the Rehmannia in the above formula is a commonly prescribed Chinese medicinal for diabetic thirst due to yin vacuity dryness.

Er Chen Wan

Er Chen Wan means Two Aged (Ingredients) Pills. This is because two of its main ingredients are aged before using. This formula is used to transform phlegm and eliminate dampness. It can be added to other appropriate formulas when phlegm dampness complicates a diabetic's Chinese pattern discrimination. Its ingredients include:

Rhizoma Pinelliae Ternatae (*Ban Xia*)
Sclerotium Poriae Cocos (*Fu Ling*)
mix-fried Radix Glycyrrhizae (*Gan Cao*)
Pericarpium Citri Reticulatae (*Chen Pi*)
uncooked Rhizoma Zingiberis (*Sheng Jiang*)

The above Chinese patent medicines only give a suggestion of how one or a combination of several over-the-counter Chinese ready-made preparations may be used to treat diabetes. As a professional practitioner of Chinese medicine, I prefer to see people receive a professional diagnosis and an individually tailored prescription. However, as long as one is careful to try to match up their pattern with the right formula and not to exceed the recommended dosages, one can try treating their diabetes with one or more of these remedies. If it works, great! These patent medicines are usually quite cheap. If this approach doesn't show any results after a couple of weeks or there are *any* side effects, one should stop taking the patent medicine and consult a professional practitioner.

Six guideposts for assessing any over-the-counter medication

In general, you can tell if any medication and treatment are good for you by checking the following six guideposts.

1. Digestion   4. Mood
2. Elimination   5. Appetite
3. Energy level   6. Sleep

If a medication, be it modern Western or traditional Chinese, gets rid of your symptoms and all six of these basic areas of human health improve, then that medicine or treatment is probably OK. However, even if a treatment or medication takes away your major complaint, if it causes deterioration in any one of these six basic parameters, then that treatment or medication is probably not OK and is certainly not OK for long-term use. When medicines and treatments, even so-called natural, herbal medications, are prescribed based on a person's pattern of disharmony, then there is healing without side effects. According to Chinese medicine, this is the only kind of true healing.

In the United States, the above Chinese patent medicines can be purchased from either of two companies which sell via the mail. Both of these companies make sincere efforts to sell only those Chinese patent medicines manufactured according to Good Manufacturing Procedures (GMP) legally imported and conforming to FDA guidelines on packaging and labeling. In addition, both these companies try not to sell medicines made from endangered species. Therefore, purchasers can feel safe that the Chinese herbal medicines purchased from these two companies are free from contamination and adulteration. Neither the author or the publishers have any business relationship with either of these two purveyors of Chinese medicinals.

Mayway Corp.
1338 Mandela Parkway Oakland, CA 94607
Tel. 510-208-3113
Orders: 1-800-MAYWAY
Fax: 510-208-3069   Orders by fax: 1-800-909-2828

Nuherbs Co.
3820 Penniman Ave.
Oakland, CA 94619
Tel. 510-534-4372
Orders: 1-800-233-4307
Fax: 510-534-4384   Orders by fax: 1-800-550-1928

Acupuncture & Moxibustion

When the average Westerner thinks of Chinese medicine, they probably first think of acupuncture. Certainly acupuncture is the best known of the various methods of treatment which go to make up Chinese medicine. However, in China, acupuncture is actually a secondary treatment modality. Most Chinese immediately think of "herbal" medicine when thinking of Chinese medicine.

Be that as it may, most professional practitioners of Chinese medicine in North America are licensed or otherwise registered and permitted to practice medicine as acupuncturists. Therefore, most such practitioners treat every patient with at least some acupuncture no matter if they also prescribe a Chinese herbal formula as well. While this "doubling up" of these two therapies is not always necessary to successfully treat most diseases, diabetic patients in general respond very well to correctly prescribed and administered acupuncture.

What is acupuncture?

Acupuncture primarily means the insertion of extremely thin, sterilized, stainless steel needles into specific points on the body where Chinese doctors have known for centuries there are special concentrations of qi and blood. Therefore, these points are like switches or circuit breakers for regulating and balancing the flow of qi and blood over the channel and network system we described above. As we have seen, diabetes is due to a breakdown in the harmony between yin and yang in the body, and, in the human body, yin and yang ultimately mean the blood and qi. As we have also seen, there really is no diabetes if there is not also spleen and stomach disharmonies causing yin and yang vacuities. A spleen and stomach disharmony means that the spleen and stomach are not fulfilling their functions of upbearing and downbearing the qi. This means that the qi is not flowing when and where it should. In addition, since the spleen governs the production of qi, blood, and body fluids, when it is weak, there is not enough qi, blood, fluids, and humors to nourish the body.

Although in China, herbal medicine is the main method of treatment for diabetes, acupuncture can be helpful as an adjunctive treatment. There are acupuncture treatment protocols for all the patterns of "flowing away and thirst" or "wasting and thirsting" described in previous chapters. In addition, acupuncture can be beneficial for treating some of the local complications of diabetes, such as vision problems, men's erectile problems, and peripheral neuropathy.

As a generic term, acupuncture also includes several other methods of stimulating acupuncture points, thus regulating the flow of qi in the body. The main other modality is moxibustion. This means the warming of acupuncture points mainly by burning dried, aged Chinese Mugwort on, near, or over acupuncture points. The purpose of this warming treatment are to 1) even more strongly stimulate the flow of qi and blood, 2) add warmth to areas of the body which are too cold, and 3) add yang qi to the body to supplement a yang qi deficiency. Other acupuncture modalities are to apply suction cups over points, to massage the points, to prick the points to allow a drop or two of blood to exit, to apply Chinese medicinals to the points, to apply magnets to the points, and to stimulate the points by either electricity or laser.

What is a typical acupuncture treatment for diabetes like?

In China, acupuncture treatments are given every day or every other day, three to five times per week depending on the nature and severity of the condition. In general, it is best if one can get acupuncture every day for the first couple of weeks if diabetes is really severe. Once the symptoms start to subside, one can begin to space out the treatments to every other day and thence to once or twice a week. However, since diabetes is a chronic, enduring disease, when acupuncture is used, it is usually done on a regular basis for extended periods of time interspersed with regular breaks.

When the person comes for their appointment, the practitioner will ask them what their main symptoms are, will typically look at their tongue and its fur, and will feel the pulses at the radial arteries on both wrists. Then, they will ask the patient to lie down on a treatment table. Based on their Chinese pattern discrimination, the practitioner will select anywhere from one to eight or nine points to be needled.

The needles used today are ethylene oxide gas sterilized disposable needles. This means that they are used one time and then thrown away, just like a hypodermic syringe in a doctor's office. However, unlike relatively fat hypodermic needles, acupuncture needles are hardly thicker than a strand of hair. The skin over the point is disinfected with alcohol and the needle is quickly and deftly inserted somewhere typically between one quarter and a half inch. In some few cases, a needle may be inserted deeper than that, but most needles are only inserted relatively shallowly.

After the needle has broken the skin, the acupuncturist will usually manipulate the needle in various ways until he or she feels that the qi has "arrived." This refers to a subtle but very real feeling of resistance around the needle. When the qi arrives, the patient will usually feel a mild, dull soreness around the needle, a slight electrical feeling, a heavy feeling, or a numb or tingly feeling. All these mean that the needle has tapped the qi and that treatment will be effective. Once the qi has been tapped, then the practitioner may further adjust the qi flow by manipulating the needle in certain ways, may attach the needle to an electro-acupuncture machine in order to stimulate the point with very mild and gentle electricity, or they may simply leave the needle in place. Usually the needles are left in place from 10-20 minutes. After this, the needles are withdrawn and thrown away. Thus there is absolutely no chance for infection from another patient.

How are the points selected?

The points that one's acupuncturist chooses to needle at each treatment are selected on the basis of Chinese medical theory and the known clinical effects of certain points. Since there are different schools or styles of acupuncture, point selection tends to vary from practitioner to practitioner. However, let me present a fairly typical case from the point of view of the dominant style of acupuncture in the People's Republic of China.

Let's say the patient's main complaints are fatigue, thirst, irritability, tightness in the chest, frontal headaches, and constipation. Their tongue is red with a thin, yellow coating. Their pulse is slightly fine, slightly rapid, and bowstring. This person's Chinese pattern discrimination is liver depression with depressive heat affecting the stomach and intestines complicated by spleen qi vacuity and fluid damage dryness. The treatment principles necessary for remedying this case are to course the liver and rectify the qi, fortify the spleen and boost the qi, clear the stomach and engender fluids. In order to accomplish these aims, the practitioner might select the following points:

Tai Chong (Liver 3)
San Yin Jiao (Spleen 6)
Zu San Li (Stomach 36)
Nei Ting (Stomach 44)
Nei Guan (Pericardium 6)
Shan Zhong (Conception Vessel 17)
He Gu (Large Intestine 4)
Zhao Hai (Kidney 6)

In this case, *Tai Chong* courses the liver and resolves depression, moves and rectifies the qi. Since liver depression qi stagnation is a factor in the disease mechanism either causing or contributing to this patient's stomach heat, this is an important point for freeing the flow of liver qi which in turn takes the wood out from under the fire of depression. In addition, this point harmonizes the liver's relationship with both the stomach and the spleen.

San Yin Jiao is a meeting place of the spleen, liver, and kidney channels. Therefore, it is chosen to further course the liver at the same time as fortifying the spleen. Its choice is like "killing two birds with one stone." Further, this point is known to promote the nourishment and supplementation of yin, blood, and body fluids, thus aiding this patient's symptoms of fluid dryness.

Zu San Li is the most powerful point on the stomach channel. Because the stomach is yang and the spleen is yin and because the stomach and spleen share a mutually "exterior/interior" relationship, stimulating *Zu San Li* can fortify the spleen with yang qi from the stomach which usually has plenty to spare. Stimulating this point can also clear heat from the stomach and harmonize the stomach. Because the stomach channel traverses the chest, needling this point can also regulate the qi in the chest, thus treating the chest tightness.

Nei Ting is another point on the stomach channel. Because it is the water point on this channel, needling it can clear heat and engender fluids within the stomach and intestines.

Nei Guan is a point on the pericardium channel which frees the flow of qi in the liver and the chest at the same time as it quiets the spirit in the heart. It also descends counterflow qi and harmonizes the stomach. Thus it treats the chest tightness and irritability at the same time as it courses the liver.

Shan Zhong is located at the level of the nipples on the chest bone between the breasts. It is a local point for freeing the flow of qi in the chest. It also upbears spleen qi and downbears stomach qi.

He Gu, a point on the large intestine channel, also upbears the clear and downbears the turbid. It frees the flow of qi in the channels, clears heat, and frees the flow of the stools. When used with *Tai Chong,* these points are called the "four bars" and strongly regulate and rectify the qi and blood of the whole body. In addition, this point is known to be very good for treating frontal headaches.

Zhao Hai is a point on the kidney channel, and although our pattern discrimination above has not mentioned anything wrong with the patient's kidneys, the kidneys are the "water viscus." This means that the kidneys are related to all yin fluids in the body, and this point is empirically known to help engender fluids. As such, it treats dry mouth and thirst above and dry stool constipation below.

Therefore, this combination of eight points addresses this patient's Chinese pattern discrimination *and* the major complaints of fatigue, thirst, irritability, tightness in the chest, frontal headache, and constipation. It remedies both the underlying disease mechanism and addresses certain key symptoms in a very direct and immediate way. Hence it provides symptomatic relief at the same time as it corrects the underlying mechanisms of these symptoms.

Does acupuncture hurt?

In Chinese, it is said that acupuncture is *bu tong*, painless. However, some patients will feel some mild soreness, heaviness, electrical tingling, or distention. Others will feel little or nothing at all. When done well and sensitively, it should not be sharp, biting, burning, or really painful.

How quickly will I feel the result?

Because irritability and nervous tension are also mostly due to liver depression qi stagnation, most people will feel an immediate relief of irritability and tension while still on the table. Typically, one will feel a pronounced tranquility and relaxation within five to ten minutes of the insertion of the needles. Many patients do drop off to sleep for a few minutes while the needles are in place.

Changes in energy level, appetite, thirst, urination, and blood sugar levels usually take several weeks of regular acupuncture before showing consistent improvements.

Who should get acupuncture?

As mentioned above, because most professional practitioners in the West are legally entitled to practice under various acupuncture laws, most acupuncturists will routinely do acupuncture on every patient. However, patients who have a lot of heat, who have a lot of qi stagnation and/or blood stasis, and patients who have bodily pain, numbness, itching, restless legs, and formication can all especially benefit from acupuncture.

When a person's diabetes mostly has to do with qi vacuity or yin vacuity, then acupuncture is not as effective as internally administered Chinese herbal medicinals. Although moxibustion can add yang qi to the body, acupuncture needles cannot add qi, blood, or yin to a body in short supply of these. The best acupuncture can do in these cases is to stimulate the various viscera and bowels which engender and transform the qi, blood, and yin. Chinese herbs, on the other hand, can directly introduce qi, blood, and yin into the body, thus supplementing vacuities and insufficiencies of these. In cases of diabetes, where qi and yin vacuities are pronounced, one should either use acupuncture *with* Chinese medicinals or rely on Chinese medicinals alone.

Ear acupuncture

Acupuncturists believe there is a map of the entire body in the ear and that by stimulating the corresponding points in the ear, one can remedy those areas and functions of the body. Therefore, many acupuncturists will not only needle points on the body at large but also select one or more points on the ear. In terms of diabetes, the points that are usually needled include Pancreas, Endocrine, Kidney, Triple Burner, Spirit Gate, Heart, and Liver. Three to five of these points are selected each session and the needles are retained for 20 minutes. This is done every other day, with 10 treatments equaling one course.

The nice thing about ear acupuncture points is that one can also use tiny "press needles" which are shaped like miniature thumbtacks. These are pressed into the points, covered with adhesive tape, and left in place for five to seven days. This method can provide continuous treatment between regularly scheduled office visits. Thus ear acupuncture is a nice way of extending the duration of an acupuncture treatment. In addition, these ear points can also be stimulated with small metal pellets, radish seeds, or tiny magnets, thus getting the benefits of stimulating these points without having to insert actual needles.

The Three Free Therapies

Although one can experiment cautiously with Chinese herbal medicinals, one cannot really do acupuncture on oneself. Therefore, Chinese herbal medicine and acupuncture and its related modalities mostly require the aid of a professional practitioner. However, there are three free therapies which are crucial to treating diabetes. These are diet, exercise, and deep relaxation. Only you can take care of these three factors in your health!

Diet

In Chinese medicine, the function of the spleen and stomach are likened to a pot on a stove or a still. The stomach receives the foods and liquids which then "rotten and ripen" like a mash in a fermentation vat. The spleen then cooks this mash and drives off (*i.e.*, transforms and upbears) the pure part. This pure or clear part collects in the lungs to become the qi and in the heart to become the blood. In addition, Chinese medicine characterizes this transformation as a process of yang qi transforming yin substance. All the principles of Chinese dietary therapy, including what persons with diabetes should and should not eat, are derived from these basic "facts."

When it comes to Chinese dietary therapy and diabetes, there are three main issues: 1) to avoid foods which lead to stomach heat, 2) to avoid foods which damage the spleen, and 3) to eat foods which help build yin and blood.

Foods which cause stomach heat

Stomach heat is probably the *sine qua non* of diabetes. If there is no stomach heat, then the lungs do not become dry above and kidney yin does not become vacuous below (at least not so vacuous as to cause serious disease). Therefore, it is important to understand what foods cause or contribute to stomach heat. These are hot, acrid, spicy foods; greasy, fatty, fried foods; and alcohol. All of these are considered warm or hot in nature according to Chinese medicine. Most people immediately understand the concept of hot, spicy foods. By hot here, I mean what in Spanish is referred to as *picante*, not *caliente*. Most food should be cooked and warm in temperature, but hot here means spicy hot like cayenne and jalapeños. But many people may not stop to consider that fatty, greasy foods include whole milk and dairy products, such as cream, butter, and cheese, and also nuts, seeds, and their resulting "butters."

As explained earlier, overeating chilled, frozen foods can cause the stomach to become overheated in a frantic effort to try and "cook" these foods into 100° soup. Stomach heat can also be the result of simply overeating. If one habitually stuffs their gullet with too much food, the stomach must also go into overdrive to deal with this. This is even more the case if one overeats or habitually eats what Chinese describe as hard to digest foods. This would include anything which is hard and tough unless very well chewed and masticated, such as hard-crusted bread or other dry, tough foods like jerky.

Foods which damage the spleen

In terms of foods which damage the spleen, Chinese medicine begins with uncooked, chilled foods. If the process of digestion is likened to cooking, then cooking is nothing other than predigestion outside of the body. In Chinese medicine, it is a given that the overwhelming majority of all food should be cooked, *i.e.*, predigested. Although cooking may destroy some vital nutrients (in Chinese, qi), cooking does render the remaining nutrients much more easily assimilable. Therefore, even though some nutrients have been lost, the net absorption of nutrients is greater with cooked foods than raw. Further, eating raw foods makes the spleen work harder and thus wears the spleen out more quickly. If one's spleen is very robust, eating uncooked, raw foods may not be so damaging, but we have already seen that many people's spleens are already weak because of their irregular eating habits and unmoderated lifestyles. It is also a fact of life that the spleen typically becomes weak with age.

More importantly, chilled foods directly damage the spleen. Chilled, frozen foods and drinks neutralize the spleen's yang qi. The process of digestion is the process of turning all foods and drinks to 100° Fahrenheit soup within the stomach so that it may undergo distillation. If the spleen expends too much yang qi just warming the food, then it will become damaged and weak even though the stomach itself may become overheated. Therefore, all foods and liquids should be eaten and drunk at room temperature at the least and better at body temperature. The more signs and symptoms of spleen vacuity a person presents, such as fatigue, chronically loose stools, undigested food in the stools, cold hands and feet, dizziness on standing up, and aversion to cold, the more closely she should avoid uncooked, chilled foods and drinks.

In addition, sugars and sweets directly damage the spleen. This is because sweet is the flavor which inherently "gathers" in the spleen. It is also an inherently dampening flavor according to Chinese medicine. This means that sweet-flavored foods if eaten to excess engender dampness internally. In Chinese medicine, it is said that the spleen is averse to dampness. Dampness is yin and controls or checks yang qi. The spleen's function is based on the transformative and transporting functions of yang qi. Therefore, anything which is excessively dampening can damage the spleen. The sweeter a food is, the more dampening and, therefore, more damaging it is to the spleen.

Another group of foods which are dampening and, therefore, damaging to the spleen is what Chinese doctors call "sodden wheat foods." This means flour products such as bread and noodles. Wheat (as opposed to rice) is damp by nature. When wheat is steamed, yeasted, and/or refined, it becomes even more dampening. In addition, all oils and fats are damp by nature and, hence, may damage the spleen. The more oily or greasy a food is, the worse it is for the spleen. Because milk contains a lot of fat, dairy products are another spleen-damaging, dampness-engendering food. Once again, this includes milk, butter, and cheese.

If we put this all together, then ice cream is just about the worst thing a person with a weak, damp spleen could eat. Ice cream is chilled, it is intensely sweet, and it is filled with fat. Therefore, it is a triple whammy when it comes to damaging the spleen and stomach. Likewise, pasta smothered in tomato sauce and cheese is a recipe for disaster. Pasta made from wheat flour is dampening, tomatoes are dampening, and cheese is dampening. In addition, what many people don't know is that a glass of fruit juice contains as much sugar as a candy bar, and, therefore, is also very damaging to the spleen and damp-engendering.

Below is a list of specific Western foods which are either uncooked, chilled, too sweet, or too dampening and thus damaging to the spleen. Persons with diabetes should minimize or avoid these proportional to how weak and damp their spleen is.

Ice cream and sugar	Juicy, sweet fruits, such as
Candy, especially chocolate	oranges, peaches, straw-
Milk	berries, and tomatoes
Butter	Fatty meats
Cheese	Fried foods
Margarine	Refined flour products
Yogurt	Yeasted bread
Raw salads	Nuts
Fruit juices	Alcohol (which is essentially
	sugar)

If the spleen is weak and wet, one should also not eat too much at any one time. A weak spleen can be overwhelmed by a large meal, especially if any of the food is difficult to digest. This then results in food stagnation which only impedes the free flow of qi all the more and further damages the spleen.

Foods which nourish yin

Most diabetics suffer from yin vacuity and fluid dryness due to long-term heat damaging and consuming yin fluids. Chinese medicine does recognize a number of foods as supplementing and enriching yin. Therefore, it would seem reasonable to suggest that people suffering from such yin and fluid vacuities eat a bunch of these yin-enriching, fluid-engendering foods.

Unfortunately, while this sounds good on paper, in practice it usually backfires. Foods which enrich yin are typically fatty, meaty foods which are not only enriching but "slimy" and hard to digest. These are so-called thick-flavored foods which are proportionally rich in turbidity. As such, these foods easily damage the spleen if eaten in excess. Since most diabetics already suffer from spleen vacuity, eating such hard-to-digest foods actually can make their situation worse.

The good news is that yin is made from qi and blood. Each day we make qi and blood from the food and liquids we take in. At the end of the day, whatever qi and blood have not been used up by our daily activities are converted into a stored form called essence. Essence is yin compared to qi which is yang. Essence can be transformed into qi, it can be transformed into blood, and it can be transformed into yin. Therefore, the really smart way to nourish yin is not to eat a whole lot of slimy, enriching, turbid, thick-flavored foods, but to eat a diet which is kind to the spleen and stomach and, therefore, promotes abundant production of qi and blood.

A clear, bland diet

In Chinese medicine, the best diet for the spleen and, therefore, by extension for most humans, is what is called a "clear, bland diet." This is a diet high in complex carbohydrates such as unrefined grains, especially rice and beans and bean products, such as tofu and tempeh. It is a diet which is high in lightly cooked vegetables. It is a diet which is low in fatty meats, oily, greasy, fried foods, and very sweet foods. However, it is not a completely or necessarily a vegetarian diet. Most people, in my experience, should eat one to two ounces of various types of meat two to four times per week. This animal flesh may be the highly popular but over-touted chicken and fish, but should also include some lean beef, pork, and lamb. Some fresh or cooked fruits may be eaten, but fruit juices should be avoided.

If the spleen is weak, then one should eat several smaller meals rather than one or two large meals. In addition, because rice is 1) neutral in temperature, 2) it fortifies the spleen and supplements the qi, and 3) it eliminates dampness, rice should be the main or staple grain in the diet. However, even when your main grain is rice, diabetics, in fact most Westerners, should not eat too many carbohydrates. While we should generally cut down on refined flour products, we should also add far more vegetables to our diets.

A few problem foods

Coffee

There are a few "problem" foods which deserve special mention. The first of these is coffee. Many people crave coffee for two reasons. First, coffee moves stuck qi. Therefore, if a person suffers from liver depression qi stagnation, temporarily coffee will make them feel like their qi is flowing. Secondly, coffee transforms essence into qi and makes that qi temporarily available to the body. Therefore, people who suffer from spleen and/or kidney vacuity fatigue will get a temporary lift from coffee. They will feel like they have energy. However, once this energy is used up, they are left with a negative deficit. The coffee has transformed some of the essence stored in the kidneys into qi. This qi has been used, and now there is less stored essence. Since the blood and essence share a common source, coffee drinking may ultimately worsen diabetes associated with blood or kidney vacuities. Tea has a similar effect as coffee in that it transforms yin essence into yang qi and liberates that upward and outward through the body. However, the caffeine in black tea is usually only half as strong as in coffee.

Chocolate

Another problem food is chocolate. Chocolate is a combination of oil, sugar, and cocoa. We have seen that both oil and sugar are dampening and damaging to the spleen. Temporarily, the sugar will boost the spleen qi, but ultimately it will result in "sugar blues" or a hypoglycemic let down. Cocoa stirs the lifegate fire. The lifegate fire is another name for kidney yang or kidney fire, and kidney fire is the source of sexual energy and desire. It is said that chocolate is the food of love, and from the Chinese medical point of view, that is true. Since chocolate stimulates kidney fire at the same time as it temporarily boosts the spleen, it does give one rush of yang qi. In addition, this rush of yang qi does move depression and stagnation, at least short-term. So it makes sense that some people with liver depression, spleen vacuity, and kidney yang debility might crave chocolate.

Alcohol

Alcohol is both damp and hot according to Chinese medical theory. Hence, in English it is referred to as "fire water." It strongly moves the qi and blood. Therefore, persons with liver depression qi stagnation will feel temporarily better from drinking alcohol. However, the sugar in alcohol damages the spleen and engenders dampness which "gums up the works," while the heat (yang) in alcohol can waste the blood (yin) and aggravate or inflame depressive liver heat and accumulated stomach heat.

105

Hot, peppery foods
Spicy, peppery, "hot" foods also move the qi, thereby giving some temporary relief to liver depression qi stagnation. However, like alcohol, the heat in spicy hot foods wastes the blood and can inflame yang.

Sour foods
In Chinese medicine, the sour flavor is inherently astringing and constricting. Therefore, people with liver depression qi stagnation should be careful not to use vinegar and other intensely sour foods. Such sour flavored foods will only aggravate the qi stagnation by astringing and restricting the qi and blood all the more. This is also why sweet and sour foods, such as orange juice and tomatoes are particularly bad for people with liver depression and spleen vacuity. The sour flavor astringes and constricts the qi, while the sweet flavor damages the spleen and engenders dampness.

Some last words on diet

In conclusion, Western patients are always asking me what they should eat in order to cure their disease. However, when it comes to diet, sad to say, the issue is not so much what to eat as what not to eat. Diet most definitely plays a major role in the cause and perpetuation of many people's diabetes, but, except in the case of vegetarians suffering from blood or yin vacuities, the issue is mainly what to avoid or minimize, not what to eat. Most of us know that coffee, chocolate, sugars and sweets, oils and fats, and alcohol are not good for us. Most of us know that we should be eating more complex carbohydrates and freshly cooked vegetables and less fatty meats. However, it's one thing to know these things and another to follow what we know.

To be perfectly honest, a clear bland diet *à la* Chinese medicine is not the most exciting diet in the world. It is the traditional diet of most lower and lower middle class peoples around the world living in temperate climates. It is the traditional diet of most of my readers' great grandparents. The point I am making here is that our modern Western diet which is high in oils and fats, high in sugars and sweets, high in animal proteins, and proportionally high in uncooked, chilled foods and drinks is a relatively recent aberration, and you can't fool Mother Nature.

When one switches to the clear, bland diet of Chinese medicine, at first one may suffer from cravings for more "flavorful" food. These cravings are, in many cases, actually associated with food "allergies." In other words, we may crave what is actually not good for us similar to a drunk who is craving alcohol. After a few days, these cravings tend to disappear and we may be amazed that we don't miss some of our convenience or "comfort" foods as much as we thought we would. If one has been addicted to a food like sugar for many years, it does not take much to "fall off the wagon" and be addicted again. Therefore, perseverance is the key to long-term success. As the Chinese say, a million is made up of nothing but lots of ones, and a bucket is quickly filled by steady drips and drops.

Exercise

Exercise is the second of what I call the three free therapies. According to Chinese medicine, regular and adequate exercise has two basic benefits. First, exercise promotes the movement of the qi and quickening of the blood. Since almost all diabetes involves at least some component of qi stagnation and blood stasis, it is obvious that exercise is an important therapy for diabetics.

Secondly, exercise benefits the spleen. The spleen's movement and transportation of the digestate is dependent upon the qi mechanism. The qi mechanism describes the function of the qi in upbearing the pure and downbearing the turbid parts of digestion. For the qi mechanism to function properly, the qi must be flowing normally and freely. Since exercise moves and rectifies the qi, it also helps regulate and rectify the qi mechanism. This then results in the spleen's movement and transportation of foods and liquids and its subsequent engendering and transforming of the qi and blood. Because spleen qi vacuity typically complicates

107

most people's diabetes and because a healthy spleen checks and controls a depressed liver, exercise treats one of the other commonly encountered disease mechanisms in the majority of Westerner's suffering from diabetes. Therefore, it is easy to see that regular, adequate exercise is a vitally important component of any person's regime for either preventing or treating diabetes.

What kind of exercise is best for diabetes?

In my experience, I find aerobic exercise to be the most beneficial for most people with diabetes. By aerobic exercise, I mean *any* physical activity which raises one's heartbeat 80% above their normal resting rate and keeps it there for at least 20 minutes. To calculate your normal resting heart rate, place your fingers over the pulsing artery on the front side of your neck. Count the beats for 15 seconds and then multiply by four. This gives you your beats per minute or BPM. Now multiply your BPM by 0.8. Take the resulting number and add it to your resting BPM. This gives you your aerobic threshold of BPM. Next engage in any physical activity you like. After you have been exercising for five minutes, take your pulse for 15 seconds once again at the artery on the front side of your throat. Again multiply the resulting count by four and this tells you your current BPM. If this number is less than your aerobic threshold BPM, then you know you need to exercise harder or faster. Once you get your heart rate up to your aerobic threshold, then you need to keep exercising at the same level of intensity for at least 20 minutes. In order to insure that one is keeping their heart beat high enough for long enough, one should recount their pulse every five minutes or so.

Depending on one's age and physical condition, different people will have to exercise harder to reach their aerobic threshold than others. For some, simply walking briskly will raise their heart beat 80% above their resting rate. For others, they will need to do calisthenics, running, swimming, racquetball, or some other, more strenuous exercise. It really does not matter what the exercise is as long as it raises your heartbeat 80% above your resting rate and keeps it there for 20 minutes.

However, there are two other criteria that should be met. One, the exercise should be something that is not too boring. If it is too boring, then you may have a hard time keeping up your schedule. Since most people do find aerobic exercises such as running, stationary bicycles, and stair-steppers boring, it is good to listen to music or watch TV in order to distract your mind from the tedium. Secondly, the type of exercise should not cause any damage to any parts of the body. For instance, running on pavement may cause knee problems for some people. Therefore, you should pick a type of exercise you enjoy but also one which will not cause any problems.

When doing aerobic exercise, it is best to exercise either every day or every other day. If one does not do their aerobics at least once every 72 hours, then its cumulative effects will not be as great. Therefore, I recommend my patients with diabetes to do some sort of aerobic exercises every day or every other day, three to four times per week at least. The good news is that there is no real need to exercise more than 30 minutes at any one time. Forty-five minutes per session is not going to be all that much better than 25 minutes per session. And 25 minutes four times per week is very much better than one hour once a week.

Deep relaxation

As we have seen above, diabetes can be associated with liver depression qi stagnation. If liver depression endures or is severe, it typically transforms into heat or fire. Heat or fire being yang, consume and exhaust yin and blood. Thus yang qi moves frenetically upward, disturbing the heart spirit. Since heat plays a pivotal role in most cases of diabetes, anything which eliminates pathological heat in the body is a good thing.

In Chinese medicine, liver depression comes from not fulfilling all one's desires. But as we have also seen above, no adult can fulfill all their desires. This is why a certain amount of liver depression is endemic among adults. When our desires are frustrated, our qi becomes depressed. This then creates emotional depression and

109

easy anger or irritability. In Chinese medicine, anger is nothing other than the venting of pent up qi in the liver. When qi becomes depressed in the liver, it accumulates like hot air in a balloon. Eventually, that hot, depressed, angry qi has to go somewhere. So when there is a little more frustration or stress, then this angry qi in the liver vents itself as irritability, anger, shouting, or nasty words, and it moves upward in the body to disturb the spirit in the heart. In Chinese medicine, it is a basic statement of fact that, "Anger results in the qi ascending."

(As an aside, it is interesting to note that, according to Chinese medicine, liver depression is also *the* root cause of an overwhelming majority of cases of hypertension or high blood pressure. Therefore, it is no surprise that many people with diabetes also have high blood pressure.)

Essentially, this type of anger and irritability are due to a maladaptive coping response that is typically learned at a young age. When we feel frustrated or stressed, stymied by or angry about something, most of us tense our muscles and especially the muscles in our upper back and shoulders, neck, and jaws. At the same time, many of us will hold our breath. This tensing of the muscles constricts the flow of qi in the channels and network vessels. Since it is the liver which is responsible for the coursing and discharging of this qi, such tensing of the muscles leads to liver depression qi stagnation. Because the lungs govern the downward spreading and movement of the qi, holding our breath due to stress or frustration only worsens this tendency of the qi not to move and, therefore, to become depressed in the Chinese medical idea of the liver.

Therefore, deep relaxation is the third of the three free therapies. For deep relaxation to be therapeutic medically, it needs to be more than just mental equilibrium. It needs to be somatic or bodily relaxation as well as mental repose. Most of us no longer recognize that every thought we think and feeling we feel is actually a felt physical sensation somewhere in our body. The words we use to describe emotions are all abstract nouns, such as anger, depression, sadness, and melancholy. However, in Chinese medicine, every emotion is associated with a change in the direction or flow of qi. As we have said above, anger makes the qi move upward. Fear, on the other hand, makes the qi move downward. Therefore, anger "makes our gorge rise" or "blow our top", while fear may cause a "sinking feeling" or make us "pee in our pants." These colloquial expressions are all based on the age-old wisdom that all thoughts and emotions are not just mental but also bodily events. This is why it is not just enough to clear one's mind. Clearing one's mind is good, but for really marked therapeutic results, it is even better if one clears one's mind at the same time as relaxing every muscle in the body.

Guided deep relaxation tapes

The single most efficient and effective way I have found for myself and my patients to practice such mental and physical deep relaxation is to do a daily, guided, progressive, deep relaxation audiotape. What I mean by guided is that a narrator on the tape leads one through the process of deep relaxation. Such tapes are progressive since they lead one through the body in a progressive manner, first relaxing one body part and then moving on to another. For instance, the narrator may say something to the effect that, as you exhale, you should feel your forehead get heavy and relaxed, softening and expanding, becoming warm and heavy. As you exhale again, now feel your cheeks get heavy and relaxed, softening and expanding, becoming warm and heavy. Breathe in and breathe out, letting your breath go without hindrance or hesitation. Breathing out, now feel your jaw muscles become heavy and relaxed, expanding and softening, becoming warm and heavy, etc., etc. throughout the entire body until one comes to the bottoms of one's feet.

There are innumerable such tapes on the market. These are usually sold in health food stores, New Age music and supply stores, or in bookstores with a good selection of New Age books. Over the years of suggesting this method of deep relaxation to my patients, I have found that each patient will have her own preferences in terms of the type of voice, male or female, the choice of words and imagery, whether there is background music or not, and the actual pace of the progression through the body, some narrators speaking a slightly different rate and rhythm. Therefore, I suggest listening to and even purchasing more than one such tape. One should find a tape which they like and can listen to without internal criticism or comment, going along like a cloud in the sky as the narrator's voice blows away all your mental and bodily stress and tension. If one has more than one tape, one can also switch every now and again from tape to tape so as not to become bored with the process or desensitized to the instructions.

Key things to look for in a good relaxation tape

In order to get the full therapeutic effect of such deep relaxation tapes, there are several key things to check for. First, be sure that the tape is a guided tape and not a subliminal relaxation tape. Subliminal tapes usually have music and any instructions to relax are given so quietly that they are not consciously heard. Although such tapes can help you feel relaxed when you do them, ultimately they do not teach you how to relax as a skill which can be consciously practiced and refined. Secondly, make sure the tape starts from the top of the body and works downward. Remember, anger makes the qi go upward in the body, and people with irritability and easy anger due to liver depression qi stagnation already have too much qi rising upward in their bodies. Such depressed qi typically needs not only to be moved but also downborne. Third, make sure the tape instructs you to relax your physical body. If you do not relax all your muscles or sinews, the qi cannot flow freely and the liver cannot be coursed. Depression is not resolved, and there will not be the same medically therapeutic effect. And lastly, be sure the tape instructs you to let your breath go with each exhalation. One of the symptoms of liver depression is a stuffy feeling in the chest which we then unconsciously try to relieve by sighing. Letting each exhalation go completely helps the lungs push the qi downward. This allows the lungs to control the liver at the same time as it downbears upwardly counterflowing angry liver qi.

The importance of daily practice

Bob Flaws, the famous American Chinese doctor, likes to tell a story about when he was an intern in Shanghai in the People's Republic of China. He was once taken on a field trip to a hospital clinic where they were using deep relaxation as a therapy with patients with high blood pressure, heart disease, stroke, migraines, and insomnia. The doctors at this clinic showed him various graphs plotting their research data on how such daily, progressive deep relaxation can regulate the blood pressure and body temperature and improve the appetite, digestion, elimination, sleep, energy, and mood. One of the things these doctors said made a big impression on Bob: "Small results in 100 days, big results in 1,000." This means that if one does such daily, progressive deep relaxation every single day for 100 days, one will definitely experience certain results. What are these "small" results? These small results are improvements in all the parameters listed above: blood pressure, body temperature, appetite, digestion, elimination, sleep, energy, and mood. If these are "small" results, then what are the "big" results experienced in 1,000 days of practice? The "big" results are a change in how one reacts to stress—in other words, a change in one's very personality or character.

What these doctors in Shanghai stressed and what I have also experienced both personally and with my patients is that it is vitally important to do such daily, guided, progressive deep relaxation every single day, day in and day out for a solid three months at least and for a continuous three years at best. If one does such progressive, somatic deep relaxation every day, one will see every parameter or measurement of health and well-being improve. If one does this kind of deep relaxation only sporadically, missing a day here and there, it will feel good when

113

you do it, but it will not have the marked, cumulative therapeutic effects it can. Therefore, perseverance is the real key to getting the benefits of deep relaxation.

The real test

Doing such a daily deep relaxation regime is like hitting tennis balls against a wall or hitting a bucket of balls at a driving range. It is only practice; it is not the real game itself. Doing a daily deep relaxation regime is not only in order to relieve one's immediate stress and strain. It is to learn a new skill, a new way to react to stress. The ultimate goal is to learn how to breathe out and immediately relax all one's muscles in the body in reaction to stress, rather than the common but unhealthy maladaption to stress of holding one's breath and tensing one's muscles. By doing such deep relaxation day after day, one learns how to relax any and every muscle in the body quickly and efficiently. Then, as soon as one recognizes they are feeling frustrated, stressed out, or uptight, they can immediately remedy those feelings at the same time as coursing their liver and rectifying their qi. This is the real test, the game of life. "Small results in 100 days, big results in 1,000."

Finding the time

If you're like me and most of my patients, you are probably asking yourself right now, "All this is well and good, but when am I supposed to find the time to eat well-balanced cooked meals, exercise at least every other day, and do a deep relaxation every day? I'm already stretched to the breaking point." I know. That's the problem.

As a clinician, I often wish I could wave a magic wand over my patients' heads and make them all healthy and well. I cannot. I know of no easy way to health. There is good living and there is easy living. Or perhaps I am stating this all wrong. What most people take as the easy way these days is to continue pushing their limits continually to the max. The so-called path of least resistance is actually the path of lots and lots of resistance. Unless you take time for yourself and find the time to eat well, exercise, and relax, no treatment is going to eliminate your diabetes completely. There is simply no pill you can pop or food you can eat that will get rid of the root causes of diabetes: poor diet, too little exercise, and too much stress.

Even Chinese herbal medicine and acupuncture can only get their full effect if the diet and lifestyle is first adjusted. Sun Si-maio, the most famous Chinese doctor of the Tang dynasty (618-907 CE), who himself refused government office and lived to be 101, said: "First adjust the diet and lifestyle and only secondarily give herbs and acupuncture." Likewise, it is said today in China, "Three parts treatment, seven parts nursing." This means that any cure is only 30% due to medical treatment and 70% is due to nursing, meaning proper diet and lifestyle.

In my experience, this is absolutely true. Seventy percent of all disease will improve after three months of proper diet, exercise, relaxation, and lifestyle modification. Seventy percent! Each of us has certain nondiscretionary rituals we perform each day. For instance, you may always and without exception find the time to brush your teeth. Perhaps it is always finding the time to shower. For others, it may be always finding the time each day to eat lunch. And for 99.999% of us, we find time, no, we *make* the time to get dressed each day. The same applies to good eating, exercise, and deep relaxation. Where there's a will there's a way. If your diabetes is bad enough, you can find the time to eat well, get proper exercise, and do a daily deep relaxation tape.

The solution to diabetes is in your hands

When I hear that patients are able to control their own conditions by following the dietary and lifestyle advice I gave them, I know that, as a Chinese doctor, I have done my job correctly. In Chinese medicine, the inferior doctor treats disease after it has appeared. The superior doctor prevents disease before it has arisen. If I can teach my patients how to cure their symptoms themselves by

115

making changes in their diet and lifestyle, then I'm approaching the goal of the high class Chinese doctor—the prevention of disease through patient education.

To get the benefits I have outline above, one must make the necessary changes in eating and behavior. In addition, diabetes is not a condition that is cured once and forever like measles or mumps. When I say Chinese medicine can cure diabetes, I do not mean that you will never experience its unwanted symptoms again. What I mean is that Chinese medicine can eliminate or greatly reduce your symptoms *as long as you keep your diet and lifestyle together.* People being people, we all "fall off the wagon" from time to time and we all "choose our own poisons." I do not expect perfection from either my patients or myself. Therefore, I am not looking for a lifetime cure. Rather, I try to give my patients an understanding of what causes their disease and what they can do to minimize or eliminate its causes and mechanisms. It is then up to the patient to decide what is bearable and what is unbearable or what is an acceptable level of health. The Chinese doctor will have done their job when you know how to correct your health to the level you find acceptable given the price you have to pay.

Simple Home Remedies for Diabetes

Since faulty diet is the main cause of diabetes, it is no wonder that most of the following Chinese home remedies for diabetes are types of Chinese dietary therapy. However, there is also a very useful Chinese self-massage regime for diabetes and a seven star hammer protocol.

Chinese medicinal porridges

Chinese medicinal porridges are a specialized part of Chinese dietary therapy. Because porridges are already in the form of 100° soup, they are a particularly good way of eating otherwise nutritious but nevertheless hard to digest grains. When Chinese medicinals are cooked along with those grains, one has a high-powered but easily assimilable "health food" of the first order.

For stomach heat accumulation and exuberance, boil 20g of Gypsum Fibrosum (*Shi Gao*) in 300ml of water for 30 minutes. Remove the dregs and reserve the liquid. Add this liquid plus another 400-600ml of plain water to 100g of polished or brown rice. Cook this into a porridge and eat each day in the morning and afternoon. Depending on how thick you like your porridge, you can cook the rice in more or less liquid. However, these porridges should all be soupy and the grains completely cooked to the point of disintegrating. Another recipe for stomach heat accumulation and exuberance is mung bean porridge. Cook 50g of mung beans with 250g of rice with as much water as you like.

Eat this one or two times per day. Mung beans clear heat, while the rice porridge engenders healthy fluids.

For stomach heat and fluid dryness, wash and cut 250g of spinach into pieces. Add this and 10g of Endothelium Corneum Gigeriae Galli (*Ji Nei Jin*) to water and cook. Then add 50g of rice and cook into mushy porridge. Eat this two times each day. Or boil 50g of uncooked Radix Rehmanniae (*Sheng Di*) and 30g of Semen Zizyphi Spinosae (*Suan Zao Ren*) in water. Remove the dregs and reserve the liquid. Then cook 100g of rice in this liquid and as much additional water as necessary to make into porridge. Eat this as you please. Yet another option is to boil 50g of watermelon seeds in water, remove the dregs, and reserve the liquid. Then cook 30g of rice in this liquid into a porridge. Also eat as you please.

For lung yin vacuity, boil 60g of Bulbus Lilii (*Bai He*) along with 100g of white rice. Eat one time each day for 10 days. Another medicinal porridge for treating lung yin vacuity diabetes can be made by cooking 60g of aduki (or azuki) beans in sufficient water to make into soup. Be sure the aduki beans are thoroughly cooked, soft and mushy. Then add 10g of Bulbus Lilii (*Bai He*) and 6g of Semen Pruni Armeniacae (*Xing Ren*) and cook for 20-30 minutes more. Eat one or more times per day.

For lung yin vacuity and spleen qi vacuity, boil 5g of Tuber Ophiopogonis Japonici (*Mai Dong*), 1.5g of Radix Panacis Ginseng (*Ren Shen*), 1.5g of Radix Glycyrrhizae (*Gan Cao*), and three pieces of Fructus Zizyphi Jujubae (*Da Zao*) in water for 20-30 minutes. Remove the dregs and reserve the liquid. Use this liquid with sufficient additional water to cook 100g of glutinous rice into porridge. Eat one or more times per day. Another recipe for lung yin vacuity with spleen qi vacuity is to cook 50g of rice into porridge. Then add 15g of sliced Rhizoma Polygonati (*Huang Jing*) and cook till the Polygonatum is tender and easily chewed. Eat this warm each morning and evening.

For lung yin vacuity, stomach yin vacuity, and stomach heat, soak 30g of Radix Trichosanthis Kirlowii (*Tian Hua Fen*) in warm water for two hours. Then add another 200ml of water and boil down till 100ml of liquid remains. Remove the dregs and reserve this liquid. Add 400ml of water to 50g of rice plus this liquid and cook into porridge. Eat two to three times per day.

For fluid dryness of the stomach and intestines with vacuity heat, cook 100g of millet into porridge with 50g of Fructus Zizyphi Jujubae (*Da Zao*) and eat occasionally.

For a combination of damp heat and stomach fluid dryness with thirst, a red tongue with scanty coating, and poor appetite, boil 20g of Fructus Pruni Mume (*Wu Mei*) in 200ml of water down to 100ml. Remove the dregs and reserve the liquid. Then add this liquid to 100g of rice and three pieces of Fructus Zizyphi Jujubae (*Da Zao*). Add another 600ml of water and cook into porridge. Eat warm each morning and evening.

For spleen qi and kidney yin vacuity, cook 30g of Tuber Asparagi Cochinensis (*Tian Men Dong*) with 50g of white rice with enough water to make a thin porridge or gruel. This porridge supplements the kidneys and enriches yin, nourishes the stomach and engenders fluids.

To supplement the lungs, spleen, and kidneys, combine 10-15g each of Radix Dioscoreae Oppositae (*Shan Yao*), Arillus Euphoriae Longanae (*Long Yan Rou*), Fructus Litchi Sinensis (*Li Zhi*), and Fructus Schizandrae Chinensis (*Wu Wei Zi*) and boil in water. Remove the dregs and reserve the liquid. Use this liquid to cook 100g of white rice, adding as much additional water as necessary.

For numerous more Chinese medicinal porridge formulas, see *The Book of Jook, Chinese Medicinal Porridges: A Healthy Alternative to the Typical Western Breakfast* written by Bob Flaws and also published by Blue Poppy Press.

Chinese medicinal teas

Chinese medicinal teas may be seen as either Chinese herbal medicine or as Chinese dietary therapy. They consist of using only one or two Chinese herbal medicinals in order to make a tea which is then drunk as one's beverage throughout the day. Such Chinese medicinal teas are usually easier to make and better tasting than multi-ingredient, professionally prescribed decoctions. They can be used as an adjunct to professional prescribed Chinese herbs or as an adjunct to acupuncture or other Chinese therapies for diabetes.

For stomach and lung heat, grind 125g of Radix Trichosanthis Kirlowii (*Tian Hua Fen*) into a coarse powder. Use 15-20g each time, steeping this in boiling water. Drink frequently throughout the day. This tea is suitable to treat excessive thirst due to heat in the stomach causing damage to lung and stomach fluids. Do not take this tea during pregnancy since this medicinal can be an abortifacient.

For yin vacuity with vexatious heat, combine Radix Glehniae Littoralis (*Sha Shen*), 15g, Tuber Ophiopogonis Japonici (*Mai Men Dong*), 15g, uncooked Radix Rehmanniae (*Sheng Di*), 15g, and Rhizoma Polygonati Odorati (*Yu Zhu*), 5g, and grind into a coarse powder. Boil a teaspoon of this powder with water and drink one cup each day. This tea boosts the stomach, engenders fluids, and stops thirst.

For excessive thirst, heat in the heart, and copious urine, combine uncooked Rhizoma Zingiberis (*Sheng Jiang*), 2 slices, 4.5g of salt, and 6g of green tea and boil together with water. Drink the resulting tea at any time. This tea clears heat and moistens dryness, engenders fluids and stops thirst.

For stomach yin vacuity, boil 50g of Fructus Pruni Mume (*Wu Mei*) in water or steep in boiling water for 10 minutes. Drink this warm as a tea at any time throughout the day. This tea engenders fluids and stops thirst.

120

For damp heat damaging stomach and lung fluids, take 20g of watermelon peel and 8g of Radix Trichosanthis Kirlowii (*Tian Hua Fen*), place in a pot, and add water. Boil for 10-15 minutes and drink the liquid as a tea throughout the day. This tea is suitable for diabetic patients with thirst and inhibited urination.

For spleen qi and kidney yin vacuity, boil 250g of Radix Dioscoreae Oppositae (*Shan Yao*)in a large pot of water for 30-45 minutes. Then drink this freely throughout the day. This tea supplements the qi, nourishes yin, and stops thirst.

For more information on Chinese medicinal teas, see Zong Xiao-fan and Gary Liscum's *Chinese Medicinal Teas: Simple, Proven, Folk Formulas for Common Diseases & Promoting Health* also published by Blue Poppy Press.

The medicinals in all the formulas in this chapter can be purchased by mail from:

China Herb Co.
165 W. Queen Lane
Philadelphia, PA 19144
Tel: 215-843-5864 Fax: 215-849-3338 Orders: 800-221-4372

They can also be purchased from either Mayway Corp. or Nuherbs Co. whose telephone and fax numbers and addresses have been given above in chapter 7.

When using any Chinese medicinal in any form, if there are any side effects, stop immediately and consult a professional practitioner of Chinese medicine.

Chinese vinegar eggs

While not a part of professional Chinese medicine, there is a Chinese folk remedy which is widely recommended for a host of various ailments. This is vinegar and eggs. I suppose this remedy is somewhat similar to the Western folk nostrum of a teaspoon of apple cider vinegar and honey each day. For diabetes, the recommendation is to take five fresh eggs and break them open, placing them in a jar, shell and all. Add 150ml of vinegar and allow this to sit for 36 hours. Then add another 250ml of vinegar. Take 15g each time each morning and evening.

Chinese Self-massage

Although proper regulation of the diet is absolutely necessary to control and reverse diabetes, Chinese self-massage can also help relieve its symptoms, prevent the disease from worsening, and regulate the internal functions of the body. In Chinese medicine, diabetes is related to heat in the lungs and/or stomach with weakness and debility of the lungs, spleen, and/or kidneys. Therefore, Chinese self-massage maneuvers for diabetes mainly aim at supplementing and regulating the functions of the lungs, spleen, stomach, and kidneys as well as clearing pathological heat from the body.

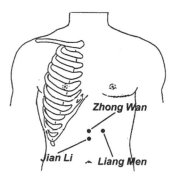

1. Press and knead *Zhong Wan* (CV 12), *Liang Men* (St 21), and *Jian Li* (CV 11): With the tip of one or both middle fingers, press and knead *Zhong Wan* (the midpoint of the upper abdomen), *Liang Men* (located 2 body inches lateral to *Zhong Wan*), and *Jian Li* (located 1 body inch below *Zhong Wan*) approximately 100 times each.

2. Rub the abdomen in a circle: With one palm, circularly rub the abdomen around the navel counter-clockwise approximately 200 times.

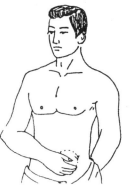

122

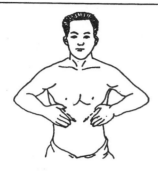

3. Straight push the abdomen: Place both palms on both sides of the abdomen. Push straight downward 30-50 times.

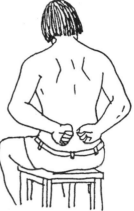

4. Press and knead the points on the back. With the bent knuckles of both thumbs, press and knead the point *Fei Shu* (Bl 13, located 1.5 body inches lateral to the lower edge of the 3rd thoracic vertebra), *Pi Shu* (Bl 20, located 1.5 body inches lateral to the lower edge of the 11th thoracic vertebra), *Wei Shu* (Bl 21, located 1.5 body inches lateral to the lower edge of the 12th thoracic vertebra), *Shen Shu* (Bl 23, located 1.5 body inches lateral to the lower edge of the 2nd lumbar vertebra), and *Yang Gang* (Bl 48, located 1.5 body inches lateral to the lower edge of the 3rd lumbar vertebra) approximately 100 times each.

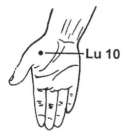

5. Press and knead *Yu Ji* (Lu 10): With the thumb of the right hand, press and knead the left *Yu Ji* (the midpoint between the base of the thumb and the base of the palm on the lateral side of the palm) 30-50 times. Then repeat this procedure on the right *Yu Ji*.

6. Press and knead *Qu Ze* (Per 3): With the tip of the middle finger or the thumb of the right hand, press and knead the left *Qu Ze* (located

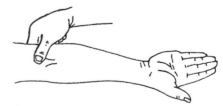

at the ulnar side of the tendon in the transverse elbow crease) 30-50 times. Then repeat this on the right *Qu Ze*.

123

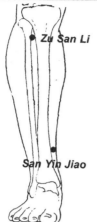

7. Press and knead *Zu San Li* (St 36): With the tips of both thumbs, press and knead *Zu San Li* (located 3 body inches below the lower outside edge of the kneecap) approximately 100 times each.

8. Press and knead *San Yin Jiao* (Sp 6): With the tips of both thumbs, press and knead the points located 3 body inches above the tip of the inner anklebones 50-100 times on each side.

Self-massage alone cannot cure or control diabetes if not supported by a clear, bland diet. For self-massage to really get its full effect, one must practice it every day for some time. When one does, one can really feel the difference it makes.

Seven star hammer

A seven star hammer is a small hammer or mallet with seven small needles embedded in its head. Nowadays in China, it is often called a skin or dermal needle. It is one of the ways a person can stimulate various acupuncture points without actually inserting a needle into the body. Seven star needles can be used either by people who are afraid of regular acupuncture, for children, or for those who wish to treat their condition at home. This technique does not need any special training or expertise. However, the protocol for diabetes will require someone to help you with the points on the back.

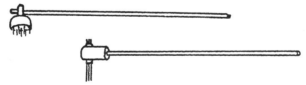

The seven star treatment of diabetes is comprised of three groups of points. Do one group of points each day, rotating through all three groups. On the first day, lightly tap both sides of the spinal

124

column, putting stress on both sides of the seventh through the 10th thoracic vertebrae. To find the seventh thoracic vertebra, find the big, knobby vertebra at the base of your neck when your head is bent forward. Then count the vertebral bumps down seven below that. That is T7. Also tap the lower edge of the jaw and the points *Zu San Li* (Stomach 36) and *He Gu* (Large Intestine 4).

Zu San Li (Stomach 36) is located three inches below the lower, outside edge of the kneecap between the two bones of the lower leg, the tibia and fibula. (See the illustration at the top of p. 124.)

He Gu is located in the center of the flesh mound between the thumb and forefinger on the back of the hand.

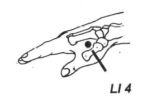

LI 4

On the second day, lightly tap the back of the neck, the sacrum, both sides of the trachea (meaning both sides of the front of the throat), the lower edge of the jaw, and the mastoid process region. The mastoid process is the bony protrusion at the base of the skull behind the ears. Then tap *Nei Guan* (Pericardium 6) and *San Yin Jiao* (Spleen 6).

Nei Guan is located three finger-widths above the crease at the palmar side of the wrist and between the two tendons.

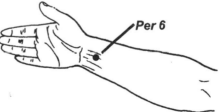

Per 6

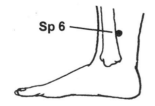

Sp 6

San Yin Jiao is located four finger-widths above the tip of the inside anklebone on the back edge of the shinbone.

On the third day, lightly tap the back of the neck, the sacrum, both sides of the seventh through the 10th thoracic vertebrae, and the points *Nei Guan* (Pericardium 6), *Zu San Li* (Stomach 36), and *Zhong Wan* (Conception Vessel 12).

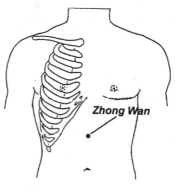

Zhong Wan is located on the midline of the stomach halfway between the bottom tip of the sternum and the belly button.

This seven star regime is also helpful for hypertension. When done regularly, it is very beneficial for diabetes. However, regularity is the key. Between treatments, soak the hammer in rubbing alcohol or hydrogen peroxide. Steven star hammers are very cheap and can be ordered from:

Oriental Medical Supply Co.
1950 Washington St., Braintree, MA 02184
Tel: (617) 331-3370 or 800-323-1839 Fax: (617) 335-5779

Kicking the Sugar Habit

Kicking a sugar habit is never easy, but, with a little willpower, it can be done. Craving sugar is an addiction like any other, and it is usually best to overcome this addiction by cutting sugar intake drastically as opposed to gradually. My suggestion is to go to your cupboard, refrigerator, and freezer and simply throw away everything in your home that has sugar in it. If you really read the labels on packaged foods, you will be shocked to learn how much of your diet has contained sugars of all kinds, some obvious, some hidden. If you have been eating a lot of sugar, you will probably feel fatigued and irritable for two to three days after you stop eating sugar. However, cravings for sugar usually stop after three days and won't come back *as long as you don't eat any sugar*. If you do, you will probably find yourself quickly addicted again.

Besides stopping eating sugar, you will also want to cut back on oils and fats and refined carbohydrates as well as on alcohol. Typically, such an overhaul of one's total diet takes one to two months to really implement such changes on a consistent basis. However, for each change you make, you should begin feeling positive effects almost immediately, and you will probably start to lose weight.

Likewise, cut out the coffee. Change to a coffee substitute made from roasted grains or dandelion roots or try Chinese green tea or Japanese bancha twig tea. Carry your tea with you in a special container or in a thermos. Then, when others are drinking coffee, you will have your tea handy. Take a good look at the coffee machine in your place of work, and you will probably see how dirty it is. If it has been cleaned, you might ask what kind of chemicals were used to clean it. Then you will know what poisons you are avoiding.

Stop drinking sodas. Here I mean both regular, sugar-filled, caffeinated sodas and also sugar-free, caffeine-free sodas. Sodas are acidic in nature and full of either sugar or chemicals. Having talked to a number of health care practitioners, we are all in agreement that even sugar-free sodas are bad for your health. Some of the symptoms caused by diet sodas in certain individuals include dribbling urination and incontinence and headaches. Who needs these? You certainly don't.

Avoid cakes, pastries, and cookies. These are made from the unholy trio of saturated fats, sugar, and refined flour. It would be hard to find a better recipe for causing diabetes than these, unless it was ice cream. Don't be misled by marketing ploys. Junk food with slick marketing is still junk food. It doesn't become less noxious because it has a hip wrapper. Check all the labels and ingredients before you indulge.

I know this is a big assignment, but the rewards are also great. During the next two months, while cutting refined sugar and flour from your daily life, pay particular attention to how you feel, how your emotions are, and how you sleep. Usually, changes this great in the diet will affect not only your physical well-being but your emotional well-being too. Typically, your sleep will become more restful and mornings brighter. Therefore, you will want to get up earlier in the mornings. Ultimately, you will have *more* energy *without* the sugar. You will also have fewer stomach upsets, less problems with ulcers, and healthier gums and teeth. Depression will leave you, allergies will lighten, you will probably have fewer colds and flu, and mosquitoes will find someone else to bite. (I'm serious!) In fact, you will also have easier menstrual periods and fewer muscle aches and pains.

If you eat a diet rich in whole grains and legumes (meaning beans and bean products), complex, unrefined carbohydrates, vegetables, and some meat, you will understand what I am talking about. Deciding to kick a sugar habit is in your hands. No one can make this decision for you, but the rewards will also be yours alone.

Chinese Medical Research on Diabetes

Considerable research has been done in the People's Republic of China on the effects of acupuncture and Chinese herbal medicine on diabetes. Usually, this research is in the form of a clinical audit. That means that a group of patients with the same diseases, patterns, or major complaints are given the same treatment for a certain period of time. After this time, the patients are counted to see how many were cured, how many got a marked effect, how many got some effect, and how many got no effect. This kind of "outcome-based research" has, up until only very recently, not been considered credible in the West where, for the last 30 years or so, the double-blind, placebo-controlled comparison study has been considered the "gold standard." However, such double-blind, placebo-controlled comparison studies are impossible to design in Chinese medicine and do not, in any case, measure effectiveness in a real-life situation.

Clinical audits, on the other hand, do measure actual clinical satisfaction of real-life patients. Such clinical audits may not exclude the patient's trust and belief in the therapist or the therapy as an important component in the result. However, real-life is not as neat and discreet as a controlled laboratory experiment. If the majority of patients are satisfied with the results of a particular treatment and there are no adverse side effects to that treatment, then that is good enough for the Chinese doctor, and, in my experience, that is also good enough for the vast majority of my patients.

Below are partial translations of several recent research articles published in Chinese medical journals on the treatment of diabetes. These research articles exemplify how Chinese medicine treats this common yet distressing complaint. I think that most persons reading these statistics would think that Chinese medicine was worth a try. Even better results can be expected when treatments are even more finely tuned to the individual patient as is the case in private practice here in the West.

"The Treatment of 26 Cases of Diabetes by the Methods of Boosting the Qi, Nourishing Yin, and Quickening the Blood" by Li Yi, *Yun Nan Zhong Yi Zhong Yao Zha Zhi (The Yunnan Journal of Chinese Medicine & Medicinals)*, 1997, #1, p. 12

Excessive thirst and hunger, profuse urination and gradual emaciation of the physical body are the primary symptoms of diabetes. In our own Chinese medicine, the symptoms of *xiao ke* (*i.e.,* wasting and thirsting) are similar [to diabetes]. In recent years, the incidence of diabetes has been more and more on the increase even among our Chinese population. The author has treated 26 cases of diabetes in the last four years with very good results as seen below.

The fasting blood sugar for most of the patients was more than 7.8 mmol/L (140mg/dl), and the urine sugar test was positive. Of the group, six were male, and 20 were female. The youngest was 38 years old, and the oldest was 68. The average age was 53 years old. The shortest duration of illness was six months; the longest was eight years. Among the 26 patients, two did not take Chinese medicinals before this audit, but used insulin instead, and, when stopping the insulin, their blood sugar levels increased.

The prescription consisted of:
uncooked Radix Rehmanniae (*Sheng Di*), 30g
Radix Dioscoreae Oppositae (*Shan Yao*), 30g

Radix Astragali Membranacei (*Huang Qi*), 30g
Radix Salviae Miltiorrhizae (*Dan Shen*), 15g
Cortex Ziziphi (*Huai Zao Pi*), 30g
Herba Dendrobii (*Shi Hu*), 15g
Rhizoma Atractylodis (*Cang Zhu*), 20g
Radix Scrophulariae Ningpoensis (*Xuan Shen*), 20g
Fructus Gardeniae Jasminoidis (*Zhi Zi*), 12g
Rhizoma Polygonati (*Huang Jing*), 20g
Endothelium Corneum Gigeriae Galli (*Ji Nei Jin*), 12g
Rhizoma Anemarrhenae Aspheloidis (*Zhi Mu*), 15g
Rhizoma Polygonati Odorati (*Yu Zhu*), 20g

For dry mouth and extreme thirst, Radix Trichosanthis Kirlowii (*Hua Fen*) and Fructus Pruni Mume (*Wu Mei*) were added. For lower burner damp heat and genital itching, Cortex Phellodendri (*Huang Bai*) was added. For copious, clear urination, Ootheca Mantidis (*Sang Piao Xiao*) and Fructus Schisandrae Chinensis (*Wu Wei Zi*) were added. For shortness of breath and disinclination to speak (due to lack of energy), Radix Pseudostellariae (*Tai Zi Shen*) and Radix Panacis Qinquifolii (*Xi Yang Shen*) were added. For low back and lower limb soreness and weakness, Cortex Eucommiae Ulmoidis (*Du Zhong*) was added. If there was unclear vision, then Scapus Et Inflorescentia Eriocaulonis Buergeriani (*Gu Jing Cao*) was added. If there was insomnia and profuse dreams, then Semen Zizyphi Spinosae (*Zao Ren*) and Caulis Polygoni Multiflori (*Ye Jiao Teng*) were added.

One packet (with the above doses) of these medicinals was boiled in water and taken every day. Two weeks constituted one course of treatment. At the same time, the patients were advised to control the amount of food eaten and to avoid acrid, peppery (*i.e.,* spicy), greasy, and sweet foods.

Patients were considered cured if their fasting blood sugar measured less than 6.7mmol/L (120mg/dl), their urine sugar test was negative, and their symptoms all disappeared. Patients were considered to have gotten a good result if their fasting blood sugar was less than 9.4mmol/L (170mg/dl), their urine sugar test was negative, and all their symptoms had improved. Patients were considered to have gotten no results if their fasting blood sugar was more than 9.4mmol/L (170mg/dl), their urine sugar was positive, and their clinical symptoms were only slightly better.

Based on the above criteria, eight cases were cured (30.77%). Fifteen cases got good results (57.69%), and three cases got no results (11.53%). Altogether, the amelioration rate was 88.64%. The shortest course of treatment was two weeks, and the longest was six weeks. The average treatment time was four weeks.

"Treating Diabetes by Boosting the Qi, Enriching Yin & Draining Fire" by Luo Shan, *Bei Jing Zhong Yi Za Zhi (The Beijing Journal of Chinese Medicine)*, 1998, #3, p. 41-42

In recent years, the author has treated 50 cases of diabetes with the methods of boosting the qi, enriching yin, and draining fire with satisfactory results as seen below.

Among these 50 cases, 31 were male and 19 were female. Two patients were 20 years of age or younger; while 38 patients were between 21-60 years of age. Another 10 patients were 60 years old or older. In 24 patients, the duration of illness was under a year. For 22 patients, the duration was 1-5 years. And in four patients, the duration of illness was more than five years.

For 11 patients, their fasting blood sugar was between 6.1-10.08mmol/L (110-190mg/dl). For 23 patients, their fasting blood sugar was between 10.09-12.32mmol/L (195-240mg/dl), and for 16 patients, their fasting blood sugar was higher than 12.32mmol/L (240mg/dl). Urine sugar tests were (++) for four patients, (+++) for 17 patients, and (++++) for 29 patients.

Eight patients also had cardiovascular disease, nine had cerebrovascular disease, two had pulmonary tuberculosis, 14 had urinary infections, five patients had boils, six had biliary infections, seven had peripheral neuritis, and seven patients had visual disturbances.

The basic prescription consisted of:
uncooked Radix Astragali Membranacei (*Huang Qi*)
Radix Dioscoreae Oppositae (*Shan Yao*)
Radix Trichosanthis Kirlowii (*Hua Fen*), 30g each
Radix Panacis Qinquifolii (*Xi Yang Shen*) or Radix
    Pseudostellariae (*Tai Zi Shen*), 10g
Rhizoma Atractylodis Macrocephalae (*Bai Zhu*)
uncooked Radix Rehmanniae (*Sheng Di*)
Radix Scrophulariae Ningpoensis (*Xuan Shen*)
Cortex Radicis Moutan (*Dan Pi*)
Tuber Ophiopogonis Japonici (*Mai Dong*)
Fructus Schisandrae Chinensis (*Wu Wei Zi*), 15g each
Fructus Corni Officinalis (*Shan Yu Rou*), 20g

In those with vexation and thirst with desire for liquids and profuse urination, a red tongue with scanty coating, rapid pulse, and other marked heat signs, Gypsum Fibrosum (*Shi Gao*), Rhizoma Anemarrhenae Aspheloidis (*Zhi Mu*), and Rhizoma Coptidis Chinensis (*Chuan Lian*) were added. For those with ravenous hunger, cooked Radix Rehmanniae (*Shu Di*) was added. For frequent, profuse, and clear urination, and other symptoms of lower burner vacuity cold, Cortex Cinnamomi Cassiae (*Rou Gui*), Radix Lateralis Praeparatus Aconiti Carmichaeli (*Fu Zi*), Radix Morindae Officinaliae (*Ba Ji*), and Ootheca Mantidis (*Sang Piao Xiao*) were added. For profuse sweating, Os Draconis (*Long Gu*) and Concha Ostreae (*Mu Li*) were added. When angina or coronary heart disease was present, then Fructus Trichosanthis Kirlowii (*Gua Lou*), Radix Pseudoginseng (*San Qi*), and Radix Salviae Miltiorrhizae (*Dan Shen*) were added. If there were accompanying infections, peripheral neuritis, and visual disturbances, these were treated with the appropriate medicinals.

All these medicinals were boiled in water and taken (in several divided doses) every day on an empty stomach. Twenty days constituted one course of treatment, and all the patients in this study adhered to an anti-diabetic diet. In addition, all these patients were required to participate in appropriate exercise and activity. The routine use of Western drugs to reduce sugar levels in the blood and urine was continued until each patient's sugar levels dropped, at which time, such drugs were discontinued. Nineteen patients recovered, 30 had some improvement, and one case got no result.

Case history: The patient was a 41 year-old female whose initial examination occurred in April 1996. The patient had been diabetic for over four years. Before enrolling in this study, she had taken various other orally administered herbal prescriptions, one after another, in an attempt to lower her blood sugar levels, but all with no good results. Therefore, she came to the author's clinic for treatment.

At the time the author first saw her, this woman's symptoms were thirst, hunger, excessive urination, emaciation, extreme exhaustion, vexation and agitation, dry stools, and lower limb numbness and lack of strength. Her tongue was red and its coating was thin, white, and dry, while her pulse was fine and rapid. Her blood sugar was 16mmol/L (280mg/dl), her urine sugar was (++++), and her urine ketones were (++).

Accordingly, the author diagnosed this patient's Chinese pattern as lung-stomach exuberant heat and added Gypsum Fibrosum (*Shi Gao*), Rhizoma Anemarrhenae Aspheloidis (*Zhi Mu*), and Rhizoma Coptidis Chinensis (*Huang Lian*) to the basic formula described above. Ten consecutive packets of these medicinals were prescribed, and, after that, all her symptoms were alleviated. There was no thirst, no red tongue, and no dry stool. However, the profuse sweating continued. Therefore, Gypsum and Anemarrhena were omitted, and Os Draconis (*Long Gu*) and Concha Ostreae (*Mu Li*) were added. Again, 10 packets were prescribed. After the second 10 packets, the patient was deemed cured. Her blood sugar was 5.8 mmol/L (<110mg/dl) and her urine sugar was (-). Then *Liu Wei Di Huang Wan* (Six Flavors Rehmannia Pill) and *Shen Ling Bai Zhu San* (Ginseng, Poria & Atractylodes Powder) were prescribed as a follow-up course of treatment. On a follow-up visit one year later, there had been no recurrence of this illness.

"Observations on the Effectiveness of Self-Composed *Jiang Tang Yin* (Lowering Sugar Drink) on the Treatment of 42 Cases of Diabetes Mellitus" by Xue Wen-sen, *Ji Lin Zhong Yi Yao (Jilin Chinese Medicine & Medicinals)*, #2, 1994, p.11-12

From March, 1984 to August, 1991, the author treated 42 cases of diabetes with self-composed *Jiang Tang Yin*. Among the 42 cases, 34 were male and eight were female. Their ages ranged from 35-63 years old. Their disease course had lasted from three months to 18 years, with the average disease course being five years. All of the patients in this study had been conclusively diagnosed as suffering from diabetes mellitus. Their abdominal cavity blood sugar levels were between 8.4-19.7mmol/L. Six cases were treated in the hospital and 36 cases were treated as out-patients.

Jiang Tang Yin consisted of:
uncooked Radix Rehmanniae (*Sheng Di*), 24g
Radix Dioscoreae Oppositae (*Shan Yao*), 24g
Fructus Lycii Chinensis (*Gou Qi Zi*), 15g
Herba Ecliptae Prostratae (*Han Lian Cao*), 30g
Radix Trichosanthis Kirlowii (*Tian Hua Fen*), 24g
Radix Scrophulariae Ningpoensis (*Xuan Shen*), 30g
Fructus Pruni Mume (*Wu Mei*), 12g
Rhizoma Polygonati (*Huang Jing*), 15g
Fructus Schisandrae Chinensis (*Wu Wei Zi*), 15g
Radix Glehniae Littoralis (*Sha Shen*), 15g
Radix Panacis Qinquifolii (*Xi Yang Shen*), 6g, or Radix
　Pseudostellariae (*Tai Zi Shen*), 30g

All these medicinals were boiled in water and taken, one packet per day.

Additions and subtractions were made to this basic prescription based on each patient's pattern discrimination. If there was dry heat and vexatious thirst, Radix Scutellariae Baicalensis (*Huang Qin*), Rhizoma Coptidis Chinensis (*Huang Lian*), and uncooked Gypsum Fibrosum (*Shi Gao*) were added. If there was polyphagia (*i.e.*, excessive eating), Rhizoma Polygonati Odorati (*Yu Zhu*) and cooked Radix Rehmanniae (*Shu Di*) were added. If there was dizziness and blurred vision, Flos Chrysanthemum Morifolii (*Ju Hua*), Radix Polygoni Multiflori (*He Shou Wu*), and Radix Ligustici Wallichii (*Chuan Xiong*) were added. If there was impotence, Rhizoma Curculiginis Orchioidis (*Xian Mao*) and Herba Epimedii (*Xian Ling Pi*) were added. If there was blood stasis, Radix Salviae Miltiorrhizae (*Dan Shen*) was added. And if there was exhaustion and fatigue with lack of strength and bodily emaciation, Radix Astragali Membranacei (*Huang Qi*) and Semen Cuscutae Chinensis (*Tu Si Zi*) were added.

Marked improvement meant that the symptoms disappeared and that the abdominal cavity blood sugar level either was normal or went down by 2.8-4.48mmol/L (50-80mg/dl). Some improvement meant that the symptoms were markedly diminished and that the abdominal cavity blood sugar levels went down by 1.68-2.80 mmol/L (30-50mg/dl). No result meant that there was no change in either symptoms or abdominal cavity blood sugar levels from before to after treatment.

Based on these criteria, 29 cases or 69% experienced marked improvement. Eight cases or 19% experienced some improvement. And five cases or 12% experienced no result. Thus the total amelioration rate was 88%.

"The Treatment of 13 Cases of Diabetic Polyneuritis with Modified *Bu Yang Huan Wu Tang* (Supplement Yang & Restore the Five [Viscera] Decoction)" by Guo Xia-xia & Liu Jia-yi, *Si Chuan Zhong Yi (Sichuan Chinese Medicine)*, #8, 1998, p. 19

Polyneuritis [or peripheral neuropathy][8] is a commonly seen complication of diabetic disease which is mostly seen in those with long-term diabetes. Its main clinical symptoms are bodily aching and pain and limb tingling and numbness. In Western medicine, it is mainly treated by sugar-lowering medicinals and B vitamins. However, the treatment results are not entirely satisfactory. The authors of this article have treated 13 cases of this condition in recent years with Chinese medicinals based on the principles of boosting the qi and nourishing yin, quickening the blood and freeing the flow of the network vessels, and the therapeutic results have been good. Their experiences are described below.

All the patients in this group were 40 years old or over. Nine were male and four were female. Five were seen as hospital in-patients and seven were out-patients. Three patients had had diabetes for two years, four for three years, and six for four or more years. The shortest incidence of neuritis was five months and the longest was two years. Eight cases experienced lower limb tingling and numbness, four cases had tingling and numbness of the four limbs, and 10 cases had bodily aching and pain. Nine cases complained of skin itching, three experienced muscular atrophy, three had lower limb water swelling or edema, and six experienced burning heat in the center of their feet. In 10 cases, tongue bodies were dark and had static spots or static macules.

---

[8] Diabetic polyneuritis and diabetic peripheral neuropathy are essentially the same condition, just different nomenclatures. Both are characterized by tingling, numbness, pain, itching, formication, and burning sensations which tend to be worse at night.

In three cases, tongue fur was scanty. The pulse was deep, fine, and choppy in nine cases and deep, fine, and rapid in four cases.

The basic formula used was modified *Bu Yang Huan Wu Tang*:
uncooked Radix Astragali Membranacei (*Huang Qi*), 30-60g
Radix Angelicae Sinensis (*Dang Gui*), 15-30g
Radix Rubrus Paeoniae Lactiflorae (*Chi Shao*), 10-15g
Semen Pruni Persicae (*Tao Ren*)
Flos Carthami Tinctorii (*Hong Hua*)
Lumbricus (*Di Long*)
Fructus Corni Officinalis (*Shan Zhu Rou*), 10g each
Caulis Milletiae Seu Spatholobi (*Ji Xue Teng*)
Radix Salviae Miltiorrhizae (*Dan Shen*)
Radix Scrophulariae Ningpoensis (*Xuan Shen*), 30g each
Radix Puerariae (*Ge Gen*), 15g

Additions & subtractions: If sugar in the urine was not lowered, 30g of Radix Trichosanthis Kirlowii (*Hua Fen*) were added. If blood sugar was relatively high, 30g of uncooked Radix Rehmanniae (*Sheng Di*) were added. If the stools were dry, 6-9g of Radix Et Rhizoma Rhei (*Da Huang*) were added. If there was edema, 30g of Sclerotium Poriae Cocos (*Yun Ling*) were added. If body pain was severe, 15g of Rhizoma Corydalis Yanhusuo (*Yuan Hu*) were added. If there was itching of the body, 15g of Fructus Kochiae Scopariae (*Di Fu Zi*) were added.

These were boiled in water and administered internally, one packet per day divided and administered in two doses.

In seven cases, the symptoms of tingling and numbness of the four limbs and bodily aching and pain disappeared. In another three cases, it was reduced; while in three cases, there was no effect. In all cases, there were varying degrees of improvement in the diabetes itself. The smallest number of packets administered was 15 and the largest was 30.

Case history: The patient was a 41 year-old male who was first examined on Apr. 4, 1992. For the past two years he had experienced polyphagia, each day eating 1.5-2kg of grain products and drinking 6,000-8,000ml of water. His urinary volume was 5,000-6,000ml per day. This was accompanied by a generalized lack of bodily strength, itching, and occasional diarrhea. In the last half year, there had been tingling and numbness in his four limbs and formication all over the skin of his body. There were also red-colored macular lumps on his chest and upper back. Occasionally he had lower limb edema. When he was admitted to the hospital his blood sugar was 16.63mmol/L, urine sugar was (++++), and ketones were (+). He was diagnosed as [suffering from] primary onset diabetes mellitus and polyneuritis. He was treated for 22 days with sugar-lowering medications, insulin, and vitamins B_1 and B_6 and his polyphagia, polydipsia, and polyuria all decreased. His blood sugar went down to 12.2mmol/L, urine sugar was (+++), and ketones were (-). However, his limb tingling and numbness and bodily aching and pain were as before.

Therefore, the insulin was stopped and the following Chinese medicinals were added: uncooked Radix Astragali Membranacei (*Huang Qi*), 45g, Radix Angelicae Sinensis (*Dang Gui*), Radix Rubrus Paeoniae Lactiflorae (*Chi Shao*), and Radix Puerariae (*Ge Gen*), 15g @, Semen Pruni Persicae (*Tao Ren*), Flos Carthami Tinctorii (*Hong Hua*), Lumbricus (*Di Long*), and Fructus Corni Officinalis (*Shan Zhu Rou*), 10g @, Caulis Milletiae Seu Spatholobi (*Ji Xue Teng*), Radix Salviae Miltiorrhizae (*Dan Shen*), Radix Scrophulariae Ningpoensis (*Xuan Shen*), Radix Trichosanthis Kirlowii (*Hua Fen*), and Sclerotium Poriae Cocos (*Yun Ling*), 30g @.

After three packets of these medicinals, the diarrhea had stopped. The above formula was administered without Poria but with 10g of Fructus Liquidambaris Taiwaniae (*Lu Lu Tong*) added. After 15 packets, the limb tingling and numbness, the bodily aching and pain, and the skin itching had all disappeared and the chest area macular lumps had receded. Blood sugar was 13mmol/L and urine sugar was (+++). On June 1, the patient was discharged from the hospital.

More Case Histories

In order to help readers get a better feel for how Chinese medicine treats diabetes, I have given below some more case histories. These are the stories of real-life people who have been treated with Chinese medicine for diabetes and have gotten a good effect. Hopefully, you will be able to see yourself and your symptoms in these stories and be encouraged to give Chinese medicine a try.

John

John was a 55 year-old engineer whose chief complaint was high blood pressure which he had had for 20 years. He also had suffered from coronary heart disease for six years and had been diabetic for three years. Although he had been taking insulin four times a day, his health still remained less than ideal. His fasting blood sugar was 230mg/dl. He complained about a stifling oppression in his chest with a suffocating sensation. With any amount of activity, the area in front of his heart became very uncomfortable. He had no bodily strength, his mouth was dry, and he was constantly thirsty. John had a ravenous hunger, frequent nighttime urination, cold lower limbs, and dry stools. His tongue was pale and dull in color, while his pulse was deep and bowstring. Therefore, his Chinese pattern was qi and yin dual vacuity with stasis obstruction of the heart vessels and ascendant liver yang. The formula he was prescribed was called *Jiang Tang Sheng Mai Tang Jia Wei* (Lower Sugar Engender the Pulse Decoction). This consisted of:

uncooked Radix Astragali Membranacei (*Huang Qi*), 30g
uncooked Radix Rehmanniae (*Sheng Di*), 30g

cooked Radix Rehmanniae (*Shu Di*), 30g
Radix Glehniae Littoralis (*Sha Shen*), 15g
Tuber Ophiopogonis Japonici (*Mai Dong*), 10g
Fructus Schisandrae Chinensis (*Wu Wei Zi*), 10g
uncooked Fructus Crataegi (*Shan Zha*), 15g
Radix Trichosanthis Kirlowii (*Tian Hua Fen*), 20g

To this basic formula the following medicinals were added: Rhizoma Atractylodis (*Cang Zhu*), Radix Scrophulariae Ningpoensis (*Yuan Shen*), Radix Puerariae (*Ge Gen*), Radix Salviae Miltiorrhizae (*Dan Shen*), Radix Dipsaci (*Chuan Duan*), Fructus Lycii Chinensis (*Gou Qi Zi*), Radix Achyranthis Bidentatae (*Niu Xi*), Ramulus Loranthi Seu Visci (*Sang Ji Sheng*), and Caulis Milletiae Seu Spatholobi (*Ji Xue Teng*).

The above Chinese medicinals were boiled in water and administered, one packet each day for two months. During this time, John was advised not to drink any alcohol and to reduce his insulin intake to three times a day. After two months on this formula, John's fasting blood sugar was 188mg/dl and his blood pressure had dropped as well. Then John changed his insulin intake to only two times per day and continued with this formula for another two months. After that, all his symptoms were gone, and his fasting blood sugar was 112mg/dl. Six months later, when seen on a follow-up visit, John's blood sugar level remained at 108mg/dl.

Mary

Mary was a 56 year-old travel agent. She was first diagnosed with diabetes over nine years ago. Since that time, her fasting blood sugar readings were sometimes as high as 300mg/dl and her urine sugar was (++++) to (+++++). She had tried using herbs and insulin at different times during the last few years, but nothing seemed to lower her blood sugar levels which remained between 130-220mg/dl. Then, during the last month, she got under more stress and, as a result, she reported that her condition had gotten worse. Her blood sugar level was 280mg/dl and urine sugar was

(+++). She was dizzy, her lower back and knees were aching and weak, and her urination was frequent and profuse. Her tongue was red with static macules, and the vessels under her tongue were purplish dark and engorged. In addition, Mary's pulse was deep, fine, and rapid. Based on all this, her Chinese pattern was categorized as kidney yin insufficiency and blood stasis. The formula prescribed was a combination of *Xue Fu Zhu Yu Tang* (Blood Mansion Dispel Stasis Decoction) and *Liu Wei Di Huang Tang* (Six Flavors Rehmannia Decoction) with additions and subtractions:

uncooked Radix Rehmanniae (*Sheng Di*), 15g
cooked Radix Rehmanniae (*Shu Di*), 15g
Radix Angelicae Sinensis (*Dang Gui*), 12g
Fructus Corni Officinalis (*Shan Yu Rou*), 12g
Cortex Radicis Moutan (*Dan Pi*), 10g
Radix Achyranthis Bidentatae (*Niu Xi*), 12g
Semen Pruni Persicae (*Tao Ren*), 9g
Flos Carthami Tinctorii (*Hong Hua*), 9g
Radix Bupleuri (*Chai Hu*), 6g
Fructus Citri Aurantii (*Zhi Ke*), 9g
Herba Ecliptae Prostratae (*Han Lian Cao*), 15g
Radix Trichosanthis Kirlowii (*Tian Hua Fen*), 15g
Tuber Ophiopogonis Japonici (*Mai Dong*), 10g

On the second visit, after seven packets of these medicinals, Mary's urine sugar had dropped to (++) and her fasting blood sugar was 210mg/dl. All her symptoms were resolved except for only a little thirst accompanied by a mild headache. Therefore, Radix Puerariae (*Ge Gen*), 20g, was added to the original formula and five more packets were prescribed.

On her third visit, all Mary's symptoms were now completely relieved. Both her blood and urine sugar levels were normal. In order to consolidate the treatment effect, *Liu Wei Di Huang Wan* and *Xue Fu Zhu Yu Tang* were continued for another 10 days, and Mary's blood and urine sugar levels remained within normal ranges.

Henry

Henry was 41 years old. He had been a diabetic for eight years. He had used blood sugar lowering medicinals and dietary control, but his urine sugar levels remained at (+) to (++). Last year, Henry noticed increasing lower limb numbness as well as a new sensation of tingling in his lower limbs. Henry's lower back and knees were burning and had a dull, aching pain. He was quite fatigued with no strength in his limbs, a dry throat, and profuse urine. The muscles in both of Henry's lower limbs were weak as were his knee reflexes. Henry had visited a neurologist for examination and was told that these symptoms indicated diabetic neuropathy. He was encouraged then to use insulin more routinely supplemented by B-complex vitamins. At the same time, Chinese medicinals were prescribed to enrich Henry's liver yin and strengthen his sinews:

Radix Bupleuri (*Chai Hu*), 20g
Radix Angelicae Sinensis (*Dang Gui*),15g
Radix Albus Paeoniae Lactiflorae (*Bai Shao*), 15g
Rhizoma Atractylodis Macrocephalae (*Bai Zhu*), 15g
Sclerotium Poriae Cocos (*Fu Ling*), 15g
Tuber Ophiopogonis Japonici (*Mai Dong*), 15g
uncooked Radix Rehmanniae (*Sheng Di*), 15g
Fructus Lycii Chinensis (*Gou Qi Zi*), 15g
Fructus Chaenomelis Lagenariae (*Mu Gua*), 15g
Radix Glehniae Littoralis (*Sha Shen*), 12g
Radix Achyranthis Bidentatae (*Niu Xi*), 15g
Caulis Milletiae Seu Spatholobi (*Ji Xue Teng*), 20g

Every day, Henry prepared and drank one packet of the above Chinese medicinals. After one month, the tingling in his lower limbs disappeared, his thirst had greatly improved, and his urination was normal. The pain in his lower back and knees had also improved, and Henry's urine sugar was (-). After taking *Dan*

Shen Pian (Salvia Tablets) and *Liu Wei Di Huang Wan* (Six Flavors Rehmannia Pills) for an additional 10 days, all of Henry's symptoms disappeared.

Alan

Alan was 50 years old and had been a diabetic for 15 years. Every day, Alan would check his urine for sugar, but he never checked his blood sugar on a regular basis. Then, during the last month, ulcers had begun to appear on both of his feet and an aching pain in his feet gradually became more and more severe. He was taking antibiotics and using a salve externally applied to the ulcerations, but the ulcers and pain just continued to get worse. Alan's urine sugar was at (+++), his fasting blood sugar was 190mg/dl, his spirit was fatigued, and there was lack of strength in his body and limbs. He had a bitter taste in his mouth, and Alan's stools were dry and difficult to pass. His tongue tip was red, while the coating was white and lacking moisture. Alan's pulse was felt to be deep. Thus, Alan's Chinese pattern was categorized as stasis and heat mutually binding, depletion of fluids, and qi vacuity. Two prescriptions were used: *Xiao Ke Tang* (Wasting & Thirsting Decoction) and *Xian Ren Huo Ming Yin* (Immortal's Life-saving Drink). The first formula consisted of:

Radix Puerariae (*Ge Gen*), 30g
uncooked Radix Rehmanniae (*Sheng Di*), 30g
Rhizoma Polygonati Odorati (*Yu Zhu*), 10g
Herba Dendrobii (*Shi Hu*), 10g
Bulbus Fritillariae Cirrhosae (*Bei Mu*), 10g
Radix Astragali Membranacei (*Huang Qi*), 15g
Fructus Pruni Mume (*Wu Mei*), 10g
Fructus Schisandrae Chinensis (*Wu Wei Zi*), 10g
Gypsum Fibrosum (*Shi Gao*), 30g

The second formula was composed of:
Flos Lonicerae Japonicae (*Jin Yin Hua*), 15g
Radix Trichosanthis Kirlowii (*Tian Hua Fen*), 15g
Bulbus Fritillariae Cirrhosae (*Bei Mu*), 10g

147

Radix Angelicae Sinensis (*Dang Gui*), 10g
Radix Rubrus Paeoniae Lactiflorae (*Chi Shao*), 10g
Resina Myrrhae (*Mo Yao*), 10g
Radix Ledebouriellae Divaricatae (*Fang Feng*), 10g
Radix Angelicae Dahuricae (*Bai Zhi*), 10g
Spina Gleditschiae Sinensis (*Zao Ci*), 10g
Radix Isatidis Seu Baphicacanthi (*Ban Lan Gen*), 30g
Flos Chrysanthemi Indici (*Ye Ju Hua*), 15g
Herba Taraxaci Mongolici Cum Radice (*Pu Gong Ying*), 15g
Radix Glycyrrhizae (*Gan Cao*), 5g

Alan took each formula every day as a water-boiled decoction for 20 days. After that, his urine sugar went to (+) and his fasting blood sugar went to 110mg/dl. The ulcers healed, and his spirit was restored. Alan was counseled about diet and lifestyle changes, and then given *Jian Pi Yi Qi Tang* (Fortify the Spleen & Boost the Qi Decoction) to regulate and stabilize his condition.

This formula consisted of:
Radix Astragali Membranacei (*Huang Qi*), 15g
Radix Pseudostellariae (*Tai Zi Shen*), 15g
Herba Agastachis Seu Pogostemi (*Huo Xiang*), 10g
Sclerotium Poriae Cocos (*Fu Ling*), 15g
Massa Medica Fermentata (*Shen Qu*), 10g
Radix Angelicae Dahuricae (*Bai Zhi*), 10g
Pericarpium Citri Reticulatae (*Chen Pi*), 10g
Rhizoma Pinelliae Ternatae (*Ban Xia*), 10g
Cortex Magnoliae Officinalis (*Hou Po*), 6g
Fructus Crataegi (*Shan Zha*), 10g
Fructus Cardamomi (*Dou Kou*), 6g
stir-fried Fructus Germinatus Oryzae Sativae (*Gu Ya*), 10g
stir-fried Fructus Germinatus Hordei Vulgaris (*Mai Ya*), 10g
Radix Glycyrrhizae (*Gan Cao*), 5g

Alan continued with 15 additional packets of these medicinals, and, on a follow-up visit six months later, none of the symptoms had returned. His blood sugar remained at 120mg/dl, and his urine sugar levels at (0) or (+).

Annette

Annette was 65 years old and overweight. She complained about her dry mouth, extreme thirst, and profuse urination. She said that she was always tired, had no strength, and had a poor appetite. Annette admitted to having very irregular and poor eating habits. Her urine sugar level was (+++) and her fasting blood sugar was 210mg/dl. Two hours after eating, Annette's blood sugar was at 250mg/dl, her cholesterol was at 250mg/dl, and her triglycerides were at 160mg/dl. Her tongue was red with a scanty, white coating, while her pulse was fine. Her Chinese pattern was yin vacuity and qi weakness. The prescription given to her consisted of:

Radix Puerariae (*Ge Gen*), 30g
uncooked Radix Rehmanniae (*Sheng Di*), 30g
Rhizoma Polygonati Odorati (*Yu Zhu*), 10g
Herba Dendrobii (*Shi Hu*), 10g
Rhizoma Anemarrhenae Aspheloidis (*Zhi Mu*), 15g
Radix Astragali Membranacei (*Huang Qi*), 15g
Fructus Pruni Mume (*Wu Mei*), 10g
Fructus Schisandrae Chinensis (*Wu Wei Zi*), 10g
Gypsum Fibrosum (*Shi Gao*), 30g
Radix Scrophulariae Ningpoensis (*Xuan Shen*), 15g

Annette was counseled on changing her dietary habits and encouraged to pay attention to exercise and relaxation. She had to be diligent about checking her urine sugars before and after meals and to look after her own health. The above Chinese herbal formula was administered each day for a month. After that, Annette's urine sugar level went down to (++) and her fasting blood sugar was lowered to 180mg/dl. Annette's mouth was not dry and she had no desire for liquids. Then the formula was changed to boost the qi and fortify the spleen:

Radix Astragali Membranacei (*Huang Qi*), 30g
Radix Pseudostellariae (*Tai Zi Shen*), 30g
Herba Agastachis Seu Pogostemi (*Huo Xiang*), 10g
Sclerotium Poriae Cocos (*Fu Ling*), 15g
Massa Medica Fermentata (*Shen Qu*), 10g
Radix Angelicae Dahuricae (*Bai Zhi*), 10g
Pericarpium Citri Reticulatae (*Chen Pi*), 10g
Rhizoma Pinelliae Ternatae (*Ban Xia*), 10g
Fructus Crataegi (*Shan Zha*), 10g
Fructus Cardamomii (*Dou Kou*), 6g
uncooked Rhizoma Zingiberis (*Sheng Jiang*), 2 pieces

Annette prepared and took this formula every day for three months. After finishing these medicinals, she found that her urine sugar level was (0) to (+) and that her fasting blood sugar was between 100-110mg/dl. These formulas together with her dietary and lifestyle changes had had a good effect on her diabetes. Therefore, to consolidate the treatment effect, Annette was given the following formula to regulate and stabilize her condition:

processed Radix Polygoni Multiflori (*Shou Wu*), 15g
Fructus Tribuli Terrestris (*Ci Ji Li*), 10g
Radix Pseudoginseng (*San Qi*), 10g
Fructus Lycii Chinensis (*Gou Qi Zi*), 10g
Radix Salviae Miltiorrhizae (*Dan Shen*), 10g
Radix Angelicae Sinensis (*Dang Gui*), 10g

Annette was determined to control her diabetes without insulin. So she continued with this formula for 80 more days. At the end of that time, her blood sugar levels remained in normal ranges, her cholesterol was lowered to 210mg/dl, and her triglycerides were lowered to 120mg/dl. Annette was very pleased to have lost some weight and was able to work once again around her home. She was also especially pleased that she was able to resume her social activities.

As the above case histories show, Chinese medicine treats the whole person. It is not just symptomatic treatment. In all the above cases, the patients not only experienced an improvement in their symptoms, but also had dramatic results in their blood and urine sugar levels. If these accompanying Western diagnostic signs had not disappeared, the Chinese doctor would have thought that the prescriptions were not correct.

Although Chinese medicine does not work immediately the way Western drugs do, it works without producing unwanted side effects. Even though it usually takes a few days to "kick in," since one's whole being feels so much better, it is usually worth the wait and perseverance. In addition, once one understands that Chinese medicine is not a symptomatic "quick fix," this motivates the person to keep on with a good diet, regular exercise, and daily deep relaxation.

Finding a Professional Practitioner of Chinese Medicine

Traditional Chinese medicine is one of the fastest growing holistic health care systems in the West today. At the present time, there are 50 colleges in the United States alone which offer three to four year training programs in acupuncture, moxibustion, Chinese herbal medicine, and Chinese medical massage. In addition, many of the graduates of these programs have done postgraduate studies at colleges and hospitals in China, Taiwan, Hong Kong, and Japan. Further, a growing number of trained Oriental medical practitioners have immigrated from China, Japan, and Korea to practice acupuncture and Chinese herbal medicine in the West.

Traditional Chinese medicine, including acupuncture, is a discreet and independent health care profession. It is not simply a technique that can easily be added to the array of techniques of some other health care profession. The study of Chinese medicine, acupuncture, and Chinese herbs is as rigorous as is the study of allopathic, chiropractic, naturopathic, or homeopathic medicine. Previous training in any one of these other systems does not automatically confer competence or knowledge in Chinese medicine. In order to get the full benefits and safety of Chinese medicine, one should seek out professionally trained and credentialed practitioners.

In the United States, recognition that acupuncture and Chinese medicine are their own independent professions has led to the creation of the National Commission for the Certification of Acupuncture & Oriental Medicine (NCCAOM). This commission has created and administers a national board examination in both acupuncture and Chinese herbal medicine in order to insure minimum levels of professional competence and safety. Those who pass the acupuncture exam append the letters Dipl. Ac. (Diplomate of Acupuncture) after their names, while those who pass the Chinese herbal exam use the letters Dipl. C.H. (Diplomate of Chinese Herbs). I recommend that persons wishing to experience the benefits of acupuncture and Chinese medicine should seek treatment in the U.S. only from those who are NCCAOM certified.

In addition, in the United States, acupuncture is a legal, independent health care profession in more than half the states. A few other states require acupuncturists to work under the supervision of MDs, while, in a number of states, acupuncture has yet to receive legal status. In states where acupuncture is licensed and regulated, the names of acupuncture practitioners can be found in the *Yellow Pages* of your local phone book or through contacting your State Department of Health, Board of Medical Examiners, or Department of Regulatory Agencies. In states without licensure, it is doubly important to seek treatment only from NCCAOM diplomates.

When seeking a qualified and knowledgeable practitioner, word of mouth referrals are important. Satisfied patients are the most reliable credential a practitioner can have. It is appropriate to ask the practitioner for references from previous patients treated for the same problem. It is best to work with a practitioner who can communicate effectively enough for you to feel understood and for the Chinese medical diagnosis and treatment plan to make sense. In all cases, a professional practitioner of Chinese medicine should be able and willing to give a written traditional Chinese diagnosis of the patient's pattern upon request.

For further information regarding the practice of Chinese medicine and acupuncture in the United States of America and for referrals to local professional associations and practitioners in the United States, prospective patients may contact:

National Commission for the Certification of Acupuncture & Oriental Medicine
11 Canal Center Plaza, Suite 300
Alexandria, VA 22314
Tel: (703) 548-9004
Fax: (703) 548-9079
Website: www.nccaom.org

The National Acupuncture & Oriental Medicine Alliance
14637 Starr Rd, SE
Olalla, WA 98357
Tel: (206) 851-6895
Fax: (206) 728-4841
Email: 76143.2061@compuserve.com

The American Association of Oriental Medicine
433 Front St.
Catasauqua, PA 18032-2506
Tel: (610) 433-2448
Fax: (610) 433-1832

Learning More About Chinese Medicine

For more information on Chinese medicine in general, see:

The Web That Has No Weaver: Understanding Chinese Medicine by Ted Kaptchuk, Congdon & Weed, NY, 1983. This is the best overall introduction to Chinese medicine for the serious lay reader. It has been a standard since it was first published over a dozen years ago and it has yet to be replaced.

Chinese Secrets of Health & Longevity by Bob Flaws, Sound True, Boulder, CO, 1996. This is a six tape audiocassette course introducing Chinese medicine to laypeople. It covers basic Chinese medical theory, Chinese dietary therapy, Chinese herbal medicine, acupuncture, *qi gong*, *feng shui*, deep relaxation, lifestyle, and more.

Fundamentals of Chinese Medicine by the East Asian Medical Studies Society, Paradigm Publications, Brookline, MA, 1985. This is a more technical introduction and overview of Chinese medicine intended for professional entry level students.

Traditional Medicine in Contemporary China by Nathan Sivin, Center for Chinese Studies, University of Michigan, Ann Arbor, 1987. This book discusses the development of Chinese medicine in China in the last half century as well as introducing the basic concepts of Chinese medical theory and practice.

In the Footsteps of the Yellow Emperor: Tracing the History of Traditional Acupuncture by Peter Eckman, Cypress Book Co., San Francisco, 1996. This book is a history of Chinese medicine and especially acupuncture. In it, the author traces how acupuncture came to Europe and America from China, Hong Kong, Taiwan, Japan, and Korea in the early and middle part of this century. Included are nontechnical discussions of basic Chinese medical theory and concepts.

Knowing Practice: The Clinical Encounter of Chinese Medicine by Judith Farquhar, Westview Press, Boulder, CO, 1994. This book is a more scholarly approach to the recent history of Chinese medicine in the People's Republic of China as well as an introduction to the basic methodology of Chinese medical practice. Although written by an academic sinologist and not a practitioner, it nonetheless contains many insightful and perceptive observations on the differences between traditional Chinese and modern Western medicines.

Imperial Secrets of Health and Longevity by Bob Flaws, Blue Poppy Press, Inc., Boulder, CO, 1994. This book includes a section on Chinese dietary therapy and generally introduces the basic concepts of good health according to Chinese medicine.

Chinese Herbal Remedies by Albert Y. Leung, Universe Books, NY, 1984. This book is about simple Chinese herbal home remedies.

Legendary Chinese Healing Herbs by Henry C. Lu, Sterling Publishing, Inc., NY, 1991. This book is a fun way to begin learning about Chinese herbal medicine. It is full of interesting and entertaining anecdotes about Chinese medicinal herbs.

The Mystery of Longevity by Liu Zheng-cai, Foreign Languages Press, Beijing, 1990. This book is also about general principles and practice promoting good health according to Chinese medicine.

For more information on Chinese dietary therapy, see:

The Tao of Healthy Eating According to Traditional Chinese Medicine by Bob Flaws, Blue Poppy Press, Inc., Boulder, CO, 1997. This book is a layperson's primer on Chinese dietary therapy. It includes detailed sections on the clear, bland diet as well as sections on chronic candidiasis, allergies, and much more.

The Book of Jook: Chinese Medicinal Porridges, A Healthy Alternative to the Typical Western Breakfast by Bob Flaws, Blue Poppy Press, Inc., Boulder, CO, 1995. This book is specifically about Chinese medicinal porridges made with very simple combinations of Chinese medicinal herbs.

Chinese Medicinal Wines & Elixirs by Bob Flaws, Blue Poppy Press, Inc., Boulder, CO, 1995. This book is a large collection of simple, one, two, and three ingredient Chinese medicinal wines which can be made at home.

Chinese Medicinal Teas: Simple, Proven Folk Formulas for Treating Disease & Promoting Health by Zong Xiao-fan & Gary Liscum, Blue Poppy Press, Inc., Boulder, CO, 1997. Like the above two books, this book is about one, two, and three ingredient Chinese medicinal teas which are easy to make and can be used at home as adjuncts to other, professionally prescribed treatments or for the promotion of health and prevention of disease.

The Tao of Nutrition by Maoshing Ni, Union of Tao and Man, Los Angeles, 1989

Harmony Rules: The Chinese Way of Health Through Food by Gary Butt & Frena Bloomfield, Samuel Weiser, Inc., York Beach, ME, 1985

Chinese System of Food Cures: Prevention & Remedies by Henry C. Lu, Sterling Publishing Co., Inc, NY, 1986

159

A Practical English-Chinese Library of Traditional Chinese Medicine: Chinese Medicated Diet ed. by Zhang En-qin, Shanghai College of Traditional Chinese Medicine Publishing House, Shanghai, 1990

Eating Your Way to Health—Dietotherapy in Traditional Chinese Medicine by Cai Jing-feng, Foreign Languages Press, Beijing, 1988

Chinese Medical Glossary

Chinese medicine is a system unto itself. Its technical terms are uniquely its own and cannot be reduced to the definitions of Western medicine without destroying the very fabric and logic of Chinese medicine. Ultimately, because Chinese medicine was created in the Chinese language, Chinese medicine is best and really only understood in that language. Nevertheless, as Westerners trying to understand Chinese medicine, we must translate the technical terms of Chinese medicine in English words. If some of these technical translations sound at first peculiar and their meaning is not immediately transparent, this is because no equivalent concepts exist in everyday English.

In the past, some Western authors have erroneously translated technical Chinese medical terms using Western medical or at least quasi-scientific words in an attempt to make this system more acceptable to Western audiences. For instance, the words tonify and sedate are commonly seen in the Western Chinese medical literature even though, in the case of sedate, its meaning is 180° opposite to the Chinese understanding of the word *xie. Xie* means to drain off something which has pooled and accumulated. That accumulation is seen as something excess which should not be lingering where it is. Because it is accumulating somewhere where it shouldn't, it is impeding and obstructing whatever should be moving to and through that area. The word sedate comes from the Latin word *sedere*, to sit. Therefore, the word sedate means to make something sit still. In English, we get the word sediment from this same root. However, the Chinese *xie* means draining off something which is sitting somewhere erroneously. Therefore, to think that one is going to sedate what is already sitting is a great mistake in understanding the clinical implication and application of this technical term.

Thus, in order, to preserve the integrity of this system while still making it intelligible to English language readers, I have appended the following glossary of Chinese medical technical terms. The terms themselves are based on Nigel Wiseman's *English-Chinese Chinese-English Dictionary of Chinese Medicine* published by the Hunan Science & Technology Press in Changsha, Hunan, People's Republic of China in 1995. Dr. Wiseman is, I believe, the greatest Western scholar in terms of the translation of Chinese medicine into English. As a Chinese reader myself, although I often find Wiseman's terms awkward sounding at first, I also think they convey most accurately the Chinese understanding and logic of these terms.

Acquired essence: Essence manufactured out of the surplus of qi and blood in turn created out of the refined essence of food and drink

Acupoints: Those places on the channels and network vessels where qi and blood tend to collect in denser concentrations, and thus those places where the qi and blood in the channels are especially available for manipulation

Acupuncture: The regulation of qi flow by the stimulation of certain points located on the channels and network vessels achieved mainly by the insertion of fine needles into these points

Ascendant hyperactivity of liver yang: Upwardly out of control counterflow of liver yang due to insufficient yin to hold it down in the lower part of the body

Blood: The red colored fluid which flows in the vessels and nourishes and constructs the tissues of the body

Blood stasis: Also called dead blood, malign blood, and dry blood, blood stasis is blood which is no longer moving through the vessels as it should. Instead it is precipitated in the vessels like silt in a river. Like silt, it then obstructs the free flow of the blood in the vessels and also impedes the production of new or fresh blood.

Blood vacuity: Insufficient blood manifesting in diminished nourishment, construction, and moistening of body tissues

Bowels: The hollow yang organs of Chinese medicine

Channels: The main routes for the distribution of qi and blood, but mainly qi

Clear: The pure or clear part of food and drink ingested which is then turned into qi and blood

Counterflow: An erroneous flow of qi, usually upward but sometimes horizontally as well

Dampness: A pathological accumulation of body fluids

Decoction: A method of administering Chinese medicinals by boiling these medicinals in water, removing the dregs, and drinking the resulting medicinal liquid

Depression: Stagnation and lack of movement, as in liver depression qi stagnation

Drain: To drain off or away some pathological qi or substance from where it is replete or excess

Essence: A stored, very potent form of substance and qi, usually yin when compared to yang qi, but can be transformed into yang qi

Five phase theory: An ancient Chinese system of correspondences dividing up all of reality into five phases of development which then mutually engender and check each other according to definite sequences

Lifegate fire: Another name for kidney yang or kidney fire, seen as the ultimate source of yang qi in the body

Moxibustion: Burning the herb Artemisia Argyium on, over, or near acupuncture points in order to add yang qi, warm cold, or promote the movement of the qi and blood

Network vessels: Small vessels which form a net-like web insuring the flow of qi and blood to all body tissues

Phlegm: A pathological accumulation of phlegm or mucus congealed from dampness or body fluids

Portals: Also called orifices, the openings of the sensory organs and the opening of the heart through which the spirit makes contact with the world outside

Qi: Activity, function, that which moves, transforms, defends, restrains, and warms

163

Qi mechanism: The process of transforming yin substance controlled and promoted by the qi, largely synonymous with the process of digestion

Qi vacuity: Insufficient qi manifesting in diminished movement, transformation, and function

Repletion: Excess or fullness, almost always pathological

Seven star hammer: A small hammer with needles embedded in its head used to stimulate acupoints without actually inserting needles

Spirit: The accumulation of qi in the heart which manifests as consciousness, sensory awareness, and mental-emotional function

Stagnation: Non-movement of the qi, lack of free flow, constraint

Supplement: To add to or augment, as in supplementing the qi, blood, yin, or yang

Turbid: The yin, impure, turbid part of food and drink which is sent downward to be excreted as waste

Vacuity: Emptiness or insufficiency, typically of qi, blood, yin, or yang

Vacuity heat: Heat due to hyperactive yang in turn due to insufficient controlling yin

Vessels: The main routes for the distribution of qi and blood, but mainly blood

Viscera: The solid yin organs of Chinese medicine

Yang: In the body, function, movement, activity, transformation

Yang vacuity: Insufficient warming and transforming function giving rise to symptoms of cold in the body

Yin: In the body, substance and nourishment

Yin vacuity: Insufficient yin substance necessary to both nourish, control, and counterbalance yang activity

Bibliography

Chinese language sources

Han Ying Chang Yong Yi Xue Ci Hui (*Chinese-English Glossary of Commonly Used Medical Terms*), Huang Xiao-kai, People's Health & Hygiene Press, Beijing, 1982

Nan Zhi Bing De Liang Fang Miao Fa (*Fine Formulas & Miraculous Methods for Difficult to Treat Diseases*), Wu Da-zhou & Ge Xiu-ke, Chinese National Medicine & Medicinal Technology Press, 1992

Nei Ke Bing Liang Fang (*Fine Formulas for Internal Medicine*), He Yuan-lin & Jiang Chang-yun, Yunnan University Press, Kunming, 1991

Shang Hai Lao Zhong Yi Jing Yan Xuan Bian (*A Selected Compilation of Shanghai Old Doctors' Experiences*), Shanghai Science & Technology Press, Shanghai, 1984

Xian Zai Nan Zhi Bing Zhong Yi Zhen Liao Xue (*A Study of Diagnosis & Treatmnet of Modern, Difficult to Treat Diseases*), Wu Jun-yu & Bai Yong-ke, Chinese Medicine Ancient Books Press, Beijing, 1993

Yan De Xin Zhen Zhi Ning Nan Bing Mi Chi (*A Secret Satchel of Yan De-xin's Diagnosis & Treatment of Knotty, Difficult to Treat Diseases*), Yan De-xin, Literary Press Publishing Co., Shanghai, 1997

Yu Xue Zheng Zhi (*Static Blood Patterns & Treatments*), Zhang Xue-wen, Shanxi Science & Technology Press, Xian, 1986

Zhen Jiu Chu Fang Xue (*A Study of Acupuncture & Moxibustion Prescriptions*), Wang Dai, Beijing Publishing Co., Beijing, 1990

Zhen Jiu Xue (A Study of Acupuncture & Moxibustion), Qiu Mao-liang *et al.*, Shanghai Science & Technology Press, Shanghai, 1985

Zhen Jiu Yi Xue (An Easy Study of Acupuncture & Moxibustion), Li Shou-xian, People's Health & Hygiene Press, Beijing, 1990

Zhong Guo Min Jian Cao Yao Fang (Chinese Folk Herbal Medicinal Formulas), Liu Guang-rui & Liu Shao-lin, Sichuan Science & Technology Press, Chengdu, 1992

Zhong Guo Zhong Yi Mi Fang Da Quan (A Great Compendium of Chinese National Chinese Medical Secret Formulas), ed. by Hu Zhao-ming, Literary Propagation Publishing Company, Shanghai, 1992

Zhong Yi Bing Yin Bing Ji Xue (A Study of Chinese Medical Disease Causes & Disease Mechanisms), Wu Dun- xu, Shanghai College of TCM Press, Shanghai, 1989

Zhong Yi Hu Li Xue (A Study of Chinese Medical Nursing), Lu Su-ying, People's Health & Hygiene Press, Beijing, 1983

Zhong Yi Lin Chuang Ge Ke (Various Clinical Specialties in Chinese Medicine), Zhang En-qin *et al.*, Shanghai College of TCM Press, Shanghai, 1990

Zhong Yi Ling Yan Fang (Efficacious Chinese Medical Formulas), Lin Bin-zhi, Science & Technology Propagation Press, Beijing, 1991

Zhong Yi Miao Yong Yu Yang Sheng (Chinese Medicine Wondrous Uses & Nourishing Life), Ni Qi-lan, Liberation Army Press, Beijing, 1993

Zhong Yi Nei Ke Lin Chuang Shou Ce (Handbook of Chinese Medicine Internal Medicine), Xia De-xin, Shanghai Science & Technology Press, Shanghai, 1989

English language sources

A Barefoot Doctor's Manual, revised & enlarged edition, Cloudburst Press, Mayne Isle, 1977

Chinese-English Terminology of Traditional Chinese Medicine, Shuai Xue-zhong *et al.*, Hunan Science & Technology Press, Changsha, 1983

Chinese-English Manual of Commonly-used Prescriptions in Traditional Chinese Medicine, Ou Ming, ed., Joint Publishing Co., Ltd., Hong Kong, 1989

Chinese Herbal Medicine: Formulas & Strategies, Dan Bensky & Randall Barolet, Eastland Press, Seattle, 1990

Chinese Herbal Medicine: Materia Medica, Dan Bensky & Andrew Gamble, second, revised edition, Eastland Press, Seattle, 1993

A Clinical Guide to Chinese Herbs and Formulae, Cheng Song-yu & Li Fei, Churchill & Livingstone, Edinburgh, 1993

A Clinical Manual of Chinese Herbal Medicine and Acupuncture, Zhou Zhong Ying & Jin Hui De, Churchill Livingstone, Edinburgh, 1997

Chinese-English Terminology of Traditional Chinese Medicine, Shuai Xue-zhong, Hunan Science & Technology Press, Changsha, 1981

A Compendium of TCM Patterns & Treatments, Bob Flaws & Daniel Finney, Blue Poppy Press, Boulder, CO, 1996

A Comprehensive Guide to Chinese Herbal Medicine, Chen Ze-lin & Chen Mei-fang, Oriental Healing Arts Institute, Long Beach, CA, 1992

English-Chinese Chinese-English Dictionary of Chinese Medicine, Nigel Wiseman, Hunan Science & Technology Press, Changsha, 1995

Fundamentals of Chinese Acupuncture, Andrew Ellis, Nigel Wiseman & Ken Boss, Paradigm Publications, Brookline, MA, 1988

Fundamentals of Chinese Medicine, Nigel Wiseman & Andrew Ellis, Paradigm Publications, Brookline, MA, 1985

Handbook of Chinese Herbs and Formulas, Him che Yeung, self-published, LA, 1985

A Handbook of Differential Diagnosis with Key Signs & Symptoms, Therapeutic Principles, and Guiding Prescriptions, Ou-yang Yi, trans. By C.S. Cheung, Harmonious Sunshine Cultural Center, SF, 1987

Oriental Materia Medica, A Concise Guide, Hong-yen Hsu, Oriental Healing Arts Institute, Long Beach, CA, 1986

Practical Therapeutics of Traditional Chinese Medicine, Yan Wu & Warren Fischer, Paradigm Publications, Brookline, MA, 1997

Practical Traditional Chinese Medicine & Pharmacology: Clinical Experiences, Shang Xian-min *et al.*, New World Press, Beijing, 1990

Practical Traditional Chinese Medicine & Pharmacology: Herbal Formulas, Geng Jun-ying, *et al.*, New World Press, Beijing, 1991

The Essential Book of Traditional Chinese Medicine, Vol. 2: Clinical Practice, Liu Yan-chi, trans. by Fang Ting-yu & Chen Lai-di, Columbia University Press, NY, 1988

The Foundations of Chinese Medicine, Giovanni Maciocia, Churchill Livingstone, Edinburgh, 1989

The Merck Manual, 15th edition, ed. by Robert Berkow, Merck Sharp & Dohme Research Laboratories, Rahway, NJ, 1987

The Practice of Chinese Medicine, Giovanni Maciocia, Churchill Livingstone, Edinburgh, 1994

The Treatise on the Spleen & Stomach, Li Dong-yuan, trans. by Yang Shou-zhong, Blue Poppy Press, Boulder, CO, 1993

The Treatment of Knotty Diseases with Chinese Acupuncture and Chinese Herbal Medicine, Shao Nian-fang, Shandong Science & Technology Press, Jinan, 1990

The Treatment of Diabetes with Traditional Chinese Medicine, Chen Jin-ding, Shandong Science & Technology Press, Jinan, 1994

The Web That Has No Weaver, Ted Kaptchuk, Congdon & Weed, NY, 1983

Traditional Medicine in Contemporary China, Nathan Sivin, University of Michigan, Ann Arbor, 1987

Zang Fu: The Organ Systems of Traditional Chinese Medicine, second edition, Jeremy Ross, Churchill Livingstone, Edinburgh, 1985

Index

A

abdominal distention 38, 57, 66
abdominal lumps and masses 61
acquired essence 162
acupoints 162, 164
acupuncture v, vi, 28, 29, 68, 72,
    91-94, 96-99, 115, 120, 124, 131,
    153-155, 157, 158, 162, 163
acupuncture & moxibustion 91
aerobic exercise 108, 109
alcohol 41, 44, 50, 93, 100, 102,
    105-107, 126, 127, 144
amenorrhea 60
American Association of Oriental
    Medicine 155
Anemarrhena & Phellodendron
    Rehmannia Pills 80
anger, easy 58, 110, 112
anxiety 4, 39, 59, 60
appetite, poor or diminished 34, 57,
    59, 86, 87, 119, 149

B

Ba Zhen Wan 86
Bai He Gu Jin Wan 77
Bai Hu Tang 79
belching 58
bleeding disorders 60
blood v, 2-6, 9-15, 18-23, 26, 28, 29,
    31-33, 35, 38-41, 43, 44, 46, 47,
    49, 50, 57-63, 68-70, 75, 79, 80,
    83-88, 91, 92, 95-97, 99, 103,
    105-107, 109, 110, 113, 132-134,
    136-141, 143-151, 162-164
Blood Mansion Dispel Stasis Pills 88
blood stasis 40, 41, 47, 49, 50, 61-63,
    75, 88, 97, 107, 138, 145, 162
body, cold 56
breast distention and pain,
    premenstrual 57, 67
breast, lumps in the 61
breath, shortness of 59, 87, 133
breathing, rapid 62
Bu Lu-ke 38

Bu Lu-nuo 38
Bu Zhong Yi Qi Wan 82
burping 58

C

carbohydrates 3, 5, 67, 104, 106,
    127, 129
cardiac distress 6
case histories 17, 143, 151
catecholamines 2
channels & network vessels 27
cheeks, flushed red 59, 80
chest, diaphragmatic oppression 62
chest and side of the rib pain 57
chest oppression 58
chill, fear of 56
Chinese patent medicines 74, 75, 85,
    88-90
chocolate 4, 102, 105, 106
Clear Dryness & Rescue the Lungs
    Decoction 75
coffee 1, 44, 45, 104-106, 127
coma 4
complexion, pale 59, 66, 86
consciousness, loss of 4
constipation 56, 66, 67, 94, 96
constipation, turns to diarrhea 66
convulsions 4
cough 16, 62, 76
craving for sweets 39, 57

D

Dan Zhi Xiao Yao Wan 84
deafness 60
deep relaxation 99, 109-115, 151,
    157
deep relaxation tapes 111, 112
diabetes, insulin-dependent 67
diabetes, non-insulin dependent 67
diarrhea, early morning 61
diet v, 4, 31, 34, 46, 50, 55, 63, 72,
    99, 103, 104, 106, 107, 115-117,
    122, 124, 127-129, 136, 148, 151,
    159, 160

169

diet, clear, bland 104, 107, 124, 159
digestion 18, 21, 26, 27, 31-33, 38,
    41, 46, 48, 89, 100, 101, 107, 113,
    163
Diplomate of Acupuncture 154
Diplomate of Chinese Herbs 154
dizziness 54, 59-61, 86, 101, 138
dizziness standing up 54, 61
dreams, excessive 58
drinking, copious 56

E

ear acupuncture 98
Eight Pearls Pills 86
elimination 89, 113
emaciation 22, 34, 132, 136, 138
endometriosis 61
energy level 89, 97
epigastric and side of the rib
    distention and pain 58
epigastrium, discomfort in the
    stomach and 58
Er Chen Tang 71
essence 9, 13, 14, 16, 31, 32, 44, 47,
    48, 103-105, 162, 163
essence, acquired 162
exercise vi, 4, 45, 46, 50, 99,
    107-109, 114, 115, 136, 149, 151
extremities, chilled 60
extremities, tingling and numbness
    of the 60
eyes, red 53, 58

F

facial complexion, red 58
fatigue 38, 46, 57, 59-61, 66, 67, 69,
    70, 72, 73, 86, 87, 94, 96, 101,
    104, 138
fatigue of the body and limbs 62
fatigue, disinclination to speak due
    to 59
feet, heat in the palms and soles of
    the 59
feverishness 62
five phase theory 43, 45, 163

flavors, five 34, 35, 38
foods, sour 106
forgetfulness 59, 60
Free & Easy Pills 83
frustration 18, 19, 32, 39, 41-43, 110

G

gallbladder 14, 25, 26, 85
generalized edema 60
Glehnia & Ophiopogon Decoction 76
glucose 2-5
glycogen 2, 3, 5
GMP 90
Good Manufacturing Procedures 90
Gui Pi Wan 87
Guo Xia-xia 139

H

hair, premature greying of the 60
headache 53-54, 60, 65, 69, 94-96,
    145
heart vi, 1, 3, 14, 15, 19, 20, 22, 23,
    25-27, 31, 34, 39, 40, 42, 43,
    46-50, 58-62, 65, 67, 68, 70, 71,
    79, 86, 87, 95, 98, 99, 108-110,
    113, 120, 135, 143, 163, 164
heart palpitations 1, 3, 19, 39, 58-61,
    65, 86, 87
heart, racing 60
heart-lung dual vacuity 59
heart-spleen dual vacuity 59
heat in the palms and soles of the
    feet 59
Heavenly Emperor Supplement the
    Heart Elixir 86
hemorrhoids 61
hiccup 58
home remedies 117, 158
hot, peppery foods 40, 106
hunger, excessive 56
hyperglycemia 2, 5
hypoglycemia v, 2-5, 38, 39, 63, 65
hypothalamus 3, 5

OTHER BOOKS ON CHINESE MEDICINE
AVAILABLE FROM BLUE POPPY PRESS
3450 Penrose Place, Suite 110, Boulder, CO 80301
For ordering 1-800-487-9296 PH. 303\447-8372 FAX 303\245-8362

A NEW AMERICAN ACUPUNC-TURE by Mark Seem, ISBN 0-936185-44-9

ACUPOINT POCKET REFERENCE ISBN 0-936185-93-7

ACUPUNCTURE AND MOXI-BUSTION FORMULAS & TREATMENTS by Cheng Dan-an, trans. by Wu Ming, ISBN 0-936185-68-6

ACUTE ABDOMINAL SYN-DROMES: Their Diagnosis & Treatment by Combined Chinese-Western Medicine by Alon Marcus, ISBN 0-936185-31-7

AGING & BLOOD STASIS: A New Approach to TCM Geriatrics by Yan De-xin, ISBN 0-936185-63-5

AIDS & ITS TREATMENT ACCORDING TO TRADI-TIONAL CHINESE MEDICINE by Huang Bing-shan, trans. by Fu-Di & Bob Flaws, ISBN 0-936185-28-7

BETTER BREAST HEALTH NATURALLY with CHINESE MEDICINE by Honora Lee Wolfe & Bob Flaws ISBN 0-936185-90-2

THE BOOK OF JOOK: Chinese Medicinal Porridges, An Alternative to the Typical Western Breakfast by B. Flaws, ISBN0-936185-60-0

CHINESE MEDICAL PALMIS-TRY: Your Health in Your Hand by Zong Xiao-fan & Gary Liscum, ISBN 0-936185-64-3

CHINESE MEDICINAL TEAS: Simple, Proven, Folk Formulas for Common Diseases & Promoting Health by Zong Xiao-fan & Gary Liscum, ISBN 0-936185-76-7

CHINESE MEDICINAL WINES & ELIXIRS by Bob Flaws, ISBN 0-936185-58-9

CHINESE PEDIATRIC MASSAGE THERAPY: A Parent's & Practitioner's Guide to the Prevention & Treatment of Childhood Illness by Fan Ya-li, ISBN 0-936185-54-6

CHINESE SELF-MASSAGE THERAPY: The Easy Way to Health by Fan Ya-li ISBN 0-936185-74-0

THE CLASSIC OF DIFFICULTIES: A Translation of the Nan Jing ISBN 1-891845-07-1

A COMPENDIUM OF TCM PAT-TERNS & TREATMENTS by Bob Flaws & Daniel Finney, ISBN 0-936185-70-8

CURING ARTHRITIS NATURALLY WITH CHINESE MEDICINE by Douglas Frank & Bob Flaws ISBN 0-936185-87-2

CURING DEPRESSION NATURALLY WITH CHINESE MEDICINE by Rosa Schnyer & Bob Flaws ISBN 0-936185-94-5

CURING HAY FEVER NATUR-ALLY WITH CHINESE MEDICINE by Bob Flaws, ISBN 0-936185-91-0

CURING HEADACHES NATURALLY WITH CHINESE MEDICINE, by Bob Flaws, ISBN 0-936185-95-3

CURING INSOMNIA NATURALLY WITH CHINESE MEDICINE by Bob Flaws ISBN 0-936185-85-6

CURING PMS NATURALLY WITH CHINESE MEDICINE by Bob Flaws ISBN 0-936185-85-6

THE DAO OF INCREASING LONGEVITY AND CONSERVING ONE'S LIFE by Anna Lin & Bob Flaws, ISBN 0-936185-24-4

A STUDY OF DAOIST ACUPUNC-TURE & MOXIBUSTION by Liu Zheng-cai ISBN 1-891845-08-X

THE DIVINE FARMER'S MAT-ERIA MEDICA (*A Translation of the Shen Nong Ben Cao*) ISBN 0-936185-96-1

THE DIVINELY RESPONDING CLASSIC: A Translation of the Shen Ying Jing from Zhen Jiu Da Cheng, trans. by Yang Shou-zhong & Liu Feng-ting ISBN 0-936185-55-4

DUI YAO: THE ART OF COMBINING CHINESE HERBAL MEDICINALS by Philippe Sionneau ISBN 0-936185-81-3

ENDOMETRIOSIS, INFERTILITY AND TRADITIONAL CHINESE MEDICINE: A Laywoman's Guide by Bob Flaws ISBN 0-936185-14-7

THE ESSENCE OF LIU FENG-WU'S GYNECOLOGY by Liu Feng-wu, translated by Yang Shou-zhong ISBN 0-936185-88-0

EXTRA TREATISES BASED ON INVESTIGATION & INQUIRY: A Translation of Zhu Dan-xi's Ge Zhi Yu Lun, by Yang & Duan, ISBN 0-936185-53-8

FIRE IN THE VALLEY: TCM Diagnosis & Treatment of Vaginal Diseases ISBN 0-936185-25-2

FU QING-ZHU'S GYNECOLOGY trans. by Yang Shou-zhong and Liu Da-wei, ISBN 0-936185-35-X

FULFILLING THE ESSENCE: A Handbook of Traditional & Contemporary Treatments for Female Infertility by Bob Flaws, ISBN 0-936185-48-1

GOLDEN NEEDLE WANG LE-TING: A 20th Century Master's Approach to Acupuncture by Yu Hui-chan and Han Fu-ru, trans. by Shuai Xue-zhong

A HANDBOOK OF TRADI-TIONAL CHINESE DERMATOL-OGY by Liang Jian-hui, trans. by Zhang & Flaws, ISBN 0-936185-07-4

A HANDBOOK OF TRADITION-AL CHINESE GYNECOLOGY by Zhejiang College of TCM, trans. by Zhang Ting-liang, ISBN 0-936185-06-6 (4th edit.)

A HANDBOOK OF MENSTRUAL DISEASES IN CHINESE MEDI-CINE by Bob Flaws ISBN 0-936185-82-1

A HANDBOOK of TCM PEDIAT-RICS by Bob Flaws, ISBN 0-936185-72-4

A HANDBOOK OF TCM UROL-OGY & MALE SEXUAL DYS-FUNCTION by Anna Lin, OMD, ISBN 0-936185-36-8

THE HEART & ESSENCE OF DAN-XI'S METHODS OF TREATMENT by Xu Dan-xi, trans. by Yang, ISBN 0-926185-49-X

THE HEART TRANSMISSION OF MEDICINE by Liu Yi-ren, trans. by Yang Shou-zhong ISBN 0-936185-83-X

HIGHLIGHTS OF ANCIENT ACUPUNCTURE PRESCRIP-TIONS trans. by Wolfe & Crescenz ISBN 0-936185-23-6

How to Have A HEALTHY PREG-NANCY, HEALTHY BIRTH with Chinese Medicine by Honora Lee Wolfe, ISBN 0-936185-40-6

HOW TO WRITE A TCM HERBAL FORMULA: A Logical Methodology for the Formulation & Administration of Chinese Herbal Medicine in Decoction by Bob Flaws, ISBN 0-936185-49-X

IMPERIAL SECRETS OF HEALTH & LONGEVITY by Bob Flaws, ISBN 0-936185-51-1

KEEPING YOUR CHILD HEAL-THY WITH CHINESE MEDI-CINE by Bob Flaws, ISBN 0-936185-71-6

THE LAKESIDE MASTER'S STUDY OF THE PULSE by Li Shi-zhen, trans. by Bob Flaws, ISBN 1-891845-01-2

Li Dong-yuan's TREATISE ON THE SPLEEN & STOMACH, A Translation of the Pi Wei Lun by Yang & Li, ISBN 0-936185-41-4

LOW BACK PAIN: Care & Pre-vention with Chinese Medicine by Douglas Frank, ISBN 0-936185-66-X

MASTER HUA'S CLASSIC OF THE CENTRAL VISCERA by Hua Tuo, ISBN 0-936185-43-0

MASTER TONG'S ACUPUNC-TURE: An Ancient Alternative Style in Modern Clinical Practice by Miriam Lee 0-926185-37-6

THE MEDICAL I CHING: Oracle of the Healer Within by Miki Shima, OMD, ISBN 0-936185-38-4

MANAGING MENOPAUSE NATURALLY with Chinese Medi-cine by Honora Lee Wolfe ISBN 0-936185-98-8

PAO ZHI: Introduction to Process-ing Chinese Medicinals to Enhance Their Therapeutic Effect, by Philippe Sionneau, ISBN 0-936185-62-1

PATH OF PREGNANCY, VOL. I, Gestational Disorders by Bob Flaws, ISBN 0-936185-39-2

PATH OF PREGNANCY, Vol. II, Postpartum Diseases by Bob Flaws. ISBN 0-936185-42-2

PEDIATRIC BRONCHITIS: Its Cause, Diagnosis & Treatment According to TCM trans. by Gao Yu-li and Bob Flaws, ISBN 0-936185-26-0

PRINCE WEN HUI'S COOK: Chinese Dietary Therapy by Bob Flaws & Honora Lee Wolfe, ISBN 0-912111-05-4, $12.95 (Published by Para-digm Press)

THE PULSE CLASSIC: A Trans-lation of the Mai Jing by Wang Shu-he, trans. by Yang Shou-zhong ISBN 0-936185-75-9

RECENT TCM RESEARCH FROM CHINA, trans. by Charles Chace & Bob Flaws, ISBN 0-936185-56-2

THE SECRET OF CHINESE PULSE DIAGNOSIS by Bob Flaws, ISBN 0-936185-67-8

SEVENTY ESSENTIAL TCM FORMULAS FOR BEGINNERS by Bob Flaws, ISBN 0-936185-59-7

SHAOLIN SECRET FORMULAS for Treatment of External Injuries, by De Chan, ISBN 0-936185-08-2

STATEMENTS OF FACT IN TRADITIONAL CHINESE MEDICINE by Bob Flaws, ISBN 0-936185-52-X

STICKING TO THE POINT 1: A Rational Methodology for the Step by Step Formulation & Administration of an Acupuncture Treatment by Bob Flaws ISBN 0-936185-17-1

STICKING TO THE POINT 2: A Study of Acupuncture & Moxibustion Formulas and Strategies by Bob Flaws ISBN 0-936185-97-X

A STUDY OF DAOIST ACUPUNCTURE by Liu Zheng-cai ISBN 1-891845-08-X

TEACH YOURSELF TO READ MODERN MEDICAL CHINESE by Bob Flaws, ISBN 0-936185-99-6

THE SYSTEMATIC CLASSIC OF ACUPUNCTURE & MOXIBUSTION (*Jia Yi Jing*) by Huang-fu Mi, trans. by Yang Shou-zhong & Charles Chace, ISBN 0-936185-29-5

THE TAO OF HEALTHY EATING ACCORDING TO CHINESE MEDICINE by Bob Flaws, ISBN 0-936185-92-9

THE TREATMENT OF DISEASE IN TCM, Vol I: Diseases of the Head & Face Including Mental/Emotional Disorders by Philippe Sionneau & Lü Gang, ISBN 0-936185-69-4

THE TREATMENT OF DISEASE IN TCM, Vol. II: Diseases of the Eyes, Ears, Nose, & Throat by Sionneau & Lü, ISBN 0-936185-69-4

THE TREATMENT OF DISEASE, Vol. III: Diseases of the Mouth, Lips, Tongue, Teeth & Gums, by Sionneau & Lü, ISBN 0-936185-79-1

THE TREATMENT OF DISEASE, Vol IV: Diseases of the Neck, Shoulders, Back, & Limbs, by Philippe Sionneau & Lü Gang, ISBN 0-936185-89-9

THE TREATMENT OF DISEASE, Vol V: Diseases of the Chest & Abdomen, by Philippe Sionneau & Lü Gang, ISBN 1-891845-02-0

THE TREATMENT OF DISEASE, Vol VI: Diseases of the Urogential System & Proctology, by Philippe Sionneau & Lü Gang, ISBN 1-891845-05-5

THE TREATMENT OF EXTERNAL DISEASES WITH ACUPUNCTURE & MOXIBUSTION by Yan Cui-lan and Zhu Yun-long, ISBN 0-936185-80-5

630 QUESTIONS & ANSWERS ABOUT CHINESE HERBAL MEDICINE: A WORKBOOK & STUDY GUIDE by Bob Flaws ISBN 1-891845-04-7

230 ESSENTIAL CHINESE MEDICINALS by Bob Flaws, ISBN 1-891845-03-9